Quick Diagnosis Diagram for Adults

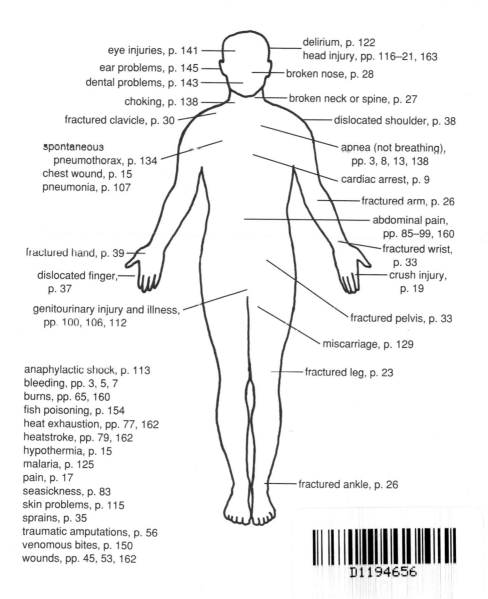

eye injuries, p. 141

ear problems, p. 145

dental problems, p. 143

choking, p. 138

fractured clavicle, p. 30

spontaneous
   pneumothorax, p. 134
chest wound, p. 15
pneumonia, p. 107

fractured hand, p. 39

dislocated finger,
   p. 37

genitourinary injury and illness,
   pp. 100, 106, 112

delirium, p. 122
head injury, pp. 116–21, 163

broken nose, p. 28

broken neck or spine, p. 27

dislocated shoulder, p. 38

apnea (not breathing),
   pp. 3, 8, 13, 138

cardiac arrest, p. 9

fractured arm, p. 26

abdominal pain,
   pp. 85–99, 160

fractured wrist,
   p. 33

crush injury,
   p. 19

fractured pelvis, p. 33

miscarriage, p. 129

fractured leg, p. 23

fractured ankle, p. 26

anaphylactic shock, p. 113
bleeding, pp. 3, 5, 7
burns, pp. 65, 160
fish poisoning, p. 154
heat exhaustion, pp. 77, 162
heatstroke, pp. 79, 162
hypothermia, p. 15
malaria, p. 125
pain, p. 17
seasickness, p. 83
skin problems, p. 115
sprains, p. 35
traumatic amputations, p. 56
venomous bites, p. 150
wounds, pp. 45, 53, 162

D1194656

Note: This diagram shows a variety of illnesses and injuries described in this book. Refer to the table of contents and the index for other ailments not listed here.

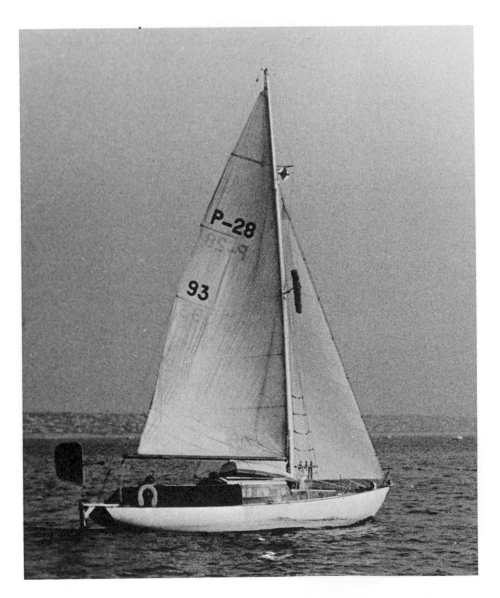

Sloop *Wa* leaving Marina del Rey, California, for an around-the-world trip.

Advanced
First Aid Afloat

FIFTH EDITION

Peter F. Eastman, M.D.
John M. Levinson, M.D., Editor

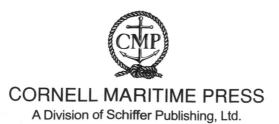

CORNELL MARITIME PRESS
A Division of Schiffer Publishing, Ltd.

To my wife Betty with great love
—P.E.

Published by Schiffer Publishing Ltd.
Advanced First Aid Afloat was originally published by Cornell Maritime Press, in 1972
Copyright © 1972 by Cornell Maritime Press
Reprint Copyright © 2010 by Schiffer Publishing Ltd.

Library of Congress Cataloging-in-Publication Data

Eastman, Peter., 1914–
    Advanced first aid afloat / Peter F. Eastman; John M. Levinson,
editor.—5th ed.
        p. cm.
    Includes index.
    ISBN 978-0-87033-524-2   (pbk.)
    1. First aid in illness and injury—Handbooks, manuals, etc.   2. Boating
injuries—Handbooks, manuals, etc.   3. Medicine,
Naval—Handbooks, manuals, etc.   I. Levinson, John M., 1927-   II. Title.
    RC88.9 .B6 E227 2000
    616.02'52'0246238—dc21   00-031589

Printed in China
First edition, 1972. Fifth edition, 2000; third printing, 2010

Schiffer Books are available at special discounts for bulk purchases for sales promotions or premiums. Special editions, including personalized covers, corporate imprints, and excerpts can be created in large quantities for special needs. For more information contact the publisher:

Published by Schiffer Publishing Ltd.
4880 Lower Valley Road
Atglen, PA 19310
Phone: (610) 593-1777; Fax: (610) 593-2002
E-mail: Info@schifferbooks.com

For the largest selection of fine reference books on this and related subjects, please visit our web site at www.schifferbooks.com
We are always looking for people to write books on new and related subjects. If you have an idea for a book please contact us at the above address.

This book may be purchased from the publisher.
Include $5.00 for shipping.
Please try your bookstore first.
You may write for a free catalog.

In Europe, Schiffer books are distributed by
Bushwood Books
6 Marksbury Ave.
Kew Gardens
Surrey TW9 4JF England
Phone: 44 (0) 20 8392-8585; Fax: 44 (0) 20 8392-9876
E-mail: info@bushwoodbooks.co.uk
Website: www.bushwoodbooks.co.uk

Contents

I. THE ADULT PATIENT

Contents

II. THE CHILD PATIENT

List of Illustrations

List of Illustrations

Preface to the Fifth Edition

In the past twenty-eight years medicine has undergone tremendous change. Much of this change is applicable to *Advanced First Aid Afloat*. First, dozens of new antibiotics are now available that were not dreamed of in 1972. Penicillin, which was efficacious for so many infections, may not be the best choice today because of resistance developed to the drug by many bacteria. Therefore, new broad-spectrum antibiotics have been incorporated in this edition offering a better chance of helping under the special conditions in which cruising sailors will be working.

Malaria treatment is constantly changing as resistance develops differently to the four types of malaria found in different regions of the world. Checking with the Centers for Disease Control (CDC) before embarking on a voyage allows one the opportunity to be properly prepared.

The communications and emergency devices now available make it far safer to obtain verbal assistance from virtually any place on the planet's vast oceans today. Besides the obligatory VHF radiophone, there are other options such as fax machines and INMARSAT satellite phone. The latter is extremely reliable but may cost $3.50 per minute of use. When your craft is in mortal danger a 406-MHz EPIRB could be lifesaving. Good communication means a cruiser can reach medical care for guidance under extreme conditions. In early 1997 during the Vendée Globe, a grueling four-month solo circumnavigation of the globe in the most dangerous of all waters, the Southern Ocean, Pete Goss on the *Aqua Quorum* was almost incapacitated by a massively swollen elbow. He was about 1,000 miles west of Cape Horn. In consultation by fax with the race surgeon and with a flashlight strapped to his head, a mirror on his knee, and a scalpel in his good hand he sliced open the massive infection. This released the pus and with antibiotics he steadily improved—and finished the race.

Before trying heroic surgery such as an amputation or even a lesser emergency, when there is time to communicate, please do so. A little advice might be lifesaving. A final plea: When you don't know what to do for your patient, do nothing. That is a most important lesson each physician or caregiver must learn.

—John M. Levinson, M.D.

Preface to the Fourth Edition

This fourth edition of *Advanced First Aid Afloat* was inspired by public acceptance of the first three editions. Time has come to bring treatment of illness and injury while cruising up to date with drugs and treatments developed in the past twenty years.

The first edition of *Advanced First Aid Afloat* was born from discussion with son Peter and his wife Addie in May 1970. They were living aboard *Wa,* their 28-foot sloop, in Santa Barbara, California, getting set to sail her around the world.

They had cruised to American Samoa in 1968 and were troubled by injury and accident that caused them much unnecessary anxiety for lack of a detailed book on extensive first aid. They asked me to help avoid this on the proposed trip.

I outlined diagnosis and treatment of common serious injury and illness in ordinary terms. They suggested revisions necessary for clearer understanding and easier use on a boat at sea.

We melded our own and many friends' relevant seafaring experiences to make this more than a dry technical manual.

Lifesaving first aid demands that three things be done quickly: Restore breathing, get the victim out of harm's way, and stop major bleeding. Bleeding is more spectacular but apnea (not breathing) is a more urgent threat to life and cannot be overlooked. Certain situations may change the order of these three actions but all three must always be considered.

When these are controlled, there is time to plan care to sustain the rescued one in good condition until he recovers or gets to a doctor.

Diagnosis and management of fractures (both simple and compound), burns, abdominal pain, genitourinary injuries, severe infections and antibiotic usage, heatstroke and exhaustion, head injury, control of irrational behavior and drugs, wounds, and serious dental problems are all discussed. Drugs and supplies relating to these subjects are presented, as well as a glossary of medical terms as used. The Introduction explains briefly how to use this book to best advantage.

Sections directed toward care of children are timely, as more and more adventurous sailors take their small offspring on long cruises. Children often present different problems in advanced first aid management even when suffering from the same illnesses and injuries that afflict adults. A child's size, together with amounts of and distribution of fluids and electrolytes, is responsible for much of this variation. In addition, children suffer a number of conditions that rarely or never involve adults.

Many people in varying fields of knowledge have helped generously in the preparation of this book. My sincere thanks go to Dr. John Pearn, professor of pediatric surgery, University of Queensland School of Medicine and the Royal Children's Hospital in Brisbane, Queensland, Australia. A recognized authority on child trauma, he was generous in the extreme with his time and knowledge to make the information accurate, timely, and well arranged.

Thanks to David B. Wallace, chemist of Mooloolaba, Queensland, Australia, for his suggestions concerning medications to have on board.

Dr. Y. Hokama, professor of pathology at the John A. Burns School of Medicine at the University of Hawaii in Honolulu, made available to me knowledge of his advanced techniques in creation of a test for the ciguatoxin causing fish poisoning. These fundamental discoveries will greatly increase the safety with which fish in the South Seas can be caught and eaten by cruising sailors and commercial fisherman as well. It is truly a great discovery, since fish are the major source of protein food in the southern Pacific islands.

Thanks go to Dr. Waldo E. Nelson, senior editor of Nelson's *Textbook of Pediatrics,* published by W. B. Saunders of Philadelphia, for permission to use charts and other materials from that excellent textbook. Dr. Brian Patten, chief of Pediatrics, Nambour General Hospital of Queensland, Australia, kindly criticized and helped in the discussion of antibiotics. Dr. Clifford Pollard, staff surgeon at Redcliffe Hospital in Queensland, Australia, furnished information about age/weight charts. Dr. James Witchall's excellent publication, *First Aid Fast and Simple,* is published by Bay Books Pty. Ltd. of New South Wales, Australia, who granted me the privilege of using some of his material in methods of taking a child's pulse.

Mr. Alan Whelpton, president of the Australian Surf Life Saving Association, granted permission to use material from a manual published by this group. Illustrations relating to cardiopulmonary resuscitation were most helpful.

My wife Betty; Ken Long of Mooloolaba, Queensland, Australia; and Marcy Dunn Ramsey made the line drawings. Thanks also to Julie Smith of Mooloolaba for her photographs. And last but very far from least, Jackie Field with her skill turned my barely legible scrawlings into attractive manuscript that anyone would be happy to send to his publisher.

Finally, there have been many who have helped along the way with true tales of their medical troubles while cruising. To all of them who remain anonymous, great thanks.

I hope you will never need the book, but that it will serve you well if you do. Happy cruising!

—Peter F. Eastman, M.D.

Introduction

HELPFUL HINTS FOR THE USE OF THIS BOOK

The book is divided into two sections to make seagoing advanced first aid complete yet simple to use.

Chapters 1 through 17 describe first aid care for adults. Chapters 18 through 23 present information for the care of sick or injured children. These later chapters were added for the increasing numbers of long-distance sailors who have youngsters below the age of twelve years in the crew. Care of the young is often more difficult for reasons explained in chapter 18.

Before the start of a cruise or race:

1. Master the gist of chapter 1, "First Things First"—If disaster strikes, there will be no time to look through the book for this information. Much of this will be useful ashore at home as well as on a cruise. It may help you sustain a life at the instant of disaster until professional medical help (doctors, paramedics, nurses) can be summoned, a life that without your knowledge and skill might well be lost.

2. Consult with your physician and pharmacist concerning supplies and drugs, some of which will be expensive and require a bit of effort. Some items will require prescriptions written by your doctor.

3. If you plan to cruise with children twelve years old or younger read chapter 18, "Care of the Sick or Injured Child," prior to departure.

If disaster strikes:

1. Open the book to the inside front and back covers. Adult and child human figures surrounded by labels will direct you quickly to cookbook-type recipes for your medical needs. The problem may be a bit different from the actual situation under your hand but the relevance will come clear with a moment's calm thought.

1

2. When matters are more under control, read on into the discussion sections of appropriate chapters. You will find certain patterns of response common to various stresses. The reason for what you did will also become clear. Your judgment grows and anxiety for the ongoing care of your patient subsides.

Many of the illustrative cases are true misadventures overcome by courageous cruising sailors, men and women alike. These will give you a more realistic idea of how things will look if someone is injured or becomes seriously ill far out from land where the whole burden of care falls on the skipper. A word of caution—this knowledge should be used only on members of your own crew when professional help is not available. Turn it over to the professionals when they arrive or you arrive at their port. In a foreign country, the physician may dress and speak differently from the doctors back home, but you are in that person's country and the physician will care for your patient to the best of his or her ability. Let him or her do so.

First Things First

Your cruising ketch is four days out of Los Angeles Harbor toward Diamond Head. At 0700 hours a sleepy helmsman invites an unintentional jibe. The boom flies across and thumps the man on watch. He slumps to the deck between the cabin trunk and the portside chain plates, unconscious and bleeding furiously from a head cut.

What do you do next, Skipper? Like most of us, you would probably be scared unless you had learned that basic lifesaving first aid is quite simple.

And that is what this chapter will show you—how simple it is: you get to work at once. When you do this, order and action supersede panic and chaos among your crew. Your injured crewman is given the best chance for quick recovery.

BASIC PRIORITIES

Any major accident anywhere, ashore or afloat, daytime or nighttime, demands attention to four basic priorities:

1. Restore breathing. Time is important since a person suffers severe brain damage after four minutes of apnea (not breathing).
2. Get the victim out of further danger.
3. Stop serious bleeding.
4. Manage the victim's pain.

Simple, isn't it, when considered in this way? Get to your injured crewman quickly. One glance assures you he is in no further danger where he is. Do not move him. It is obvious he is bleeding; ignore that for the moment. A person can often bleed quite a while without much danger.

Note that his chest is not moving in and out; his lips, fingertips, and cheeks are blue-gray. He isn't breathing.

MOUTH-TO-MOUTH RESUSCITATION

Start mouth-to-mouth resuscitation at once (see figure 1).

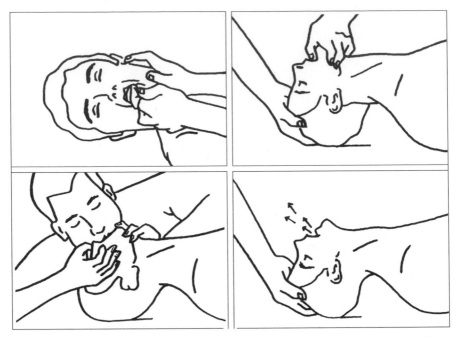

Fig.1. *Top left,* Sweep mouth clear. *Top right,* Elevate chin. *Bottom left,* Close patient's nose and, mouth-to-mouth, blow into lungs. (Note: The operator's right hand should be holding the patient's nose.) *Bottom right,* Allow free expiration.

1. Put on surgical gloves if you have them. Sweep his mouth and throat clear of blood, dentures, water—anything that obstructs the flow of air into his lungs.
2. Elevate his chin.
3. Close his nose with your thumb and forefinger.
4. Insert a resuscitating tube into his mouth. This is a plastic airway tube; one end goes into the patient's mouth, and you blow on the other (see figure 2). Use of a resuscitating tube reduces the chances of contracting an infectious disease from the victim, and its use is considered mandatory in first aid courses taught in the United States. You will need to make your own decision regarding administering mouth-to-mouth resuscitation without a resuscitating tube, knowing that the patient may not survive if you do not.
5. Take a big breath through your nose; gently blow it into the tube and down into his lungs. His chest will rise as you do this.
6. Take your mouth away; he will exhale automatically.
7. When his lungs have pushed out all the air you blew in, give him another breath.

8. Repeat this twelve to fifteen times a minute (twenty to twenty-five times a minute for a child).
9. Do not stop until his breathing is regular. He may start suddenly or with a series of irregular gasps. If he gasps, time your efforts between them. Let him do as much as he can, but keep assisting him until he is breathing well. How will you know? A ruddy glow will replace the blue-gray color on his lips and earlobes.
10. Stop then; but don't leave him unattended for the next twelve hours. Have someone stand by to assist him if he stops breathing again. This is most important if he is unconscious.

Your crew will be close about you and their hurt buddy and they will be greatly impressed with your prompt recognition that he was not breathing (some people think a person is dead if he is not breathing) and your skill at resuscitation. They will be standing by for your directions.

Detail someone steady to stop the bleeding from his head. Tell that person what to do between breaths as you keep up the mouth-to-mouth resuscitation. Forget about bleeding points, pressure points, and such detailed anatomy. Tell him to put on gloves (if available) and press down hard on whatever is bleeding. If one finger will serve—fine; if the wound is larger, he or she may need to use the whole hand. If it is bigger than that, have him or her stuff a gauze bandage, towel (preferably clean), or whatever is handy into the wound and apply the pressure over this.

You will be too busy to tell your helper this, but you know that arterial blood pressure is rarely higher than 200 mm of mercury; even a child can press harder than that. Direct pressure is what surgeons use in the operating room to stop bleeding.

Have the crew member watch the blood ooze between his or her fingers. It slows down before it stops. Keep the pressure on ten minutes longer, then have a second crew member (who has gotten out the first-aid kit) put a tight bandage around the cut head. Chances are pretty good by this time (ten minutes after you began mouth-to-mouth and five minutes after your helper bandaged the head) that your victim is breathing on his own.

He is "coming to," dazed but conscious. Left unattended and apneic (not breathing) while his head was bandaged, he might never have made it. But he has, thanks to your skill and knowledge.

Now you have leisure to plan. You surely won't leave him lying there on the deck. Why not get him below to his bunk? There may be other injuries that passed unnoted in the rush to revive him. Sailors are a sturdy breed. He may insist, "I'm all right now," and try to get to his feet unaided.

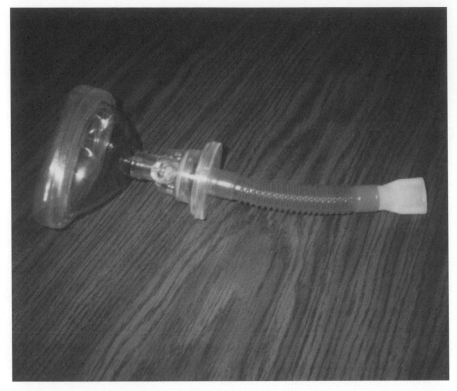

Fig. 2. Resuscitating tube.

Assert your authority—make him stay put. It is most embarrassing, and occurs in hospitals all the time, to overlook injuries other than the obvious ones that attracted your attention at the time of the accident. The results of such neglect may be disastrous.

You must know how badly he is hurt. Has he any hidden injury? How far away is medical help? Will you need such help or can you handle this yourself?

We will assume he had a complete physical checkup by his physician before departure. Therefore, he has no chronic diseases that he and you do not know about.

PHYSICAL EXAMINATION

To examine him:

1. Start at the top. He is conscious, so ask him where it hurts. His head is pretty well covered by the bandage.

2. Shine a bright flashlight into his eyes, one at a time. The pupils should be equal, and each should contract, or narrow. Unequal pupils, or one that does not contract with the light, indicate a brain concussion of a serious nature. (We will talk about head injuries and management of the unconscious patient later on.)
3. Gently move his neck; feel the entire length of his spine with your fingertips, from the base of his skull right down to, and including, his tailbone. Extreme tenderness or soreness should make you suspect a spinal injury.
4. Ask him to take a deep breath. A sharp pain in his chest may mean broken ribs. Press hard on the breastbone with your right hand and the mid-back behind it with your left. This will cause pain at the site of a broken rib, just as pressure on opposite sides of a barrel springs the hoops.
5. Feel his abdomen gently with the flat of your hand. He may have internal injuries that won't be evident for several hours, but if his abdominal wall muscles are contracted hard, and he cannot relax them when you ask him to, he probably has some such injury.
6. Finally, have him move all fingers, toes, both hands, feet, ankles, wrists, arms, legs, elbows, knees, shoulders, and hips. Note if any of these hurt or are deformed or lying at an odd angle.
7. Finally you conclude:
    a. There is no serious brain damage. He is conscious, alert, knows the day of the week, where he is, and is well oriented. His eye pupils are equal and contract alike.
    b. Findings 3, 4, 5, and 6 above are within normal limits.
    c. To the best of your knowledge he has a cut head and that is all.

Discussion

While the rest of the crew are putting the injured person in a bunk, let us consider some of the commonsense and physiological reasons behind what you have done and also some other catastrophes which can switch the order of the basic priorities. All the priorities must be considered in any major accident but judgment is necessary to determine the order in which they are carried out.

Sometimes getting a victim away from further danger is first. If electrocution is the cause of apnea, as it may well be, do not begin mouth-to-mouth resuscitation until you get the current off, or you may join the casualty list, too.

If a severe gash cuts the brachial artery (to the arm), and the victim's life is squirting away in a series of violent red gushes, the thing to do, of course, is to get a tourniquet around the arm just above the cut and twist it down until it stops the bleeding. But be sure it is spurting arterial bleeding. Look very carefully—a little blood is awesome. The usual wound will not sever a main artery; the bleeding will be a mixture of small arterial and venous bleeding, and pressure followed by bandaging will stop it.

If you decide on a tourniquet, twist it tight enough. Pad it well. Use a piece of line, a belt, anything sturdy enough to lay about the limb and twist tight. Every twenty minutes you must loosen a tourniquet long enough to make the limb below feel warm and alive again, even if the bleeding resumes while it is loosened. We will say more about the follow-up care of wounds in chapter 3.

Consider a more complicated situation. You are dismasted; one of the crew is overside in a tangle of lines and stays. He is obviously in danger and must be freed up and rescued. But is he breathing? If you spend fifteen minutes or more cutting him loose and he has been apneic all that time . . . ? If he answers your holler, you know he is conscious and breathing. But if he does not, get to him on a lifeline or other rig and resuscitate him while somebody else frees him up and brings him aboard. You will both remember this with gratitude in years to come.

Many injuries produce apnea. A blow on the head, such as we have discussed, may so stun the brain that it stops driving the respiratory muscles in their proper cycles. This may be temporary; the brain may recover with a good supply of oxygen. But that is just what the non-breathing person will not get without assistance. Four minutes is the upper limit of apnea without severe brain damage or even death.

Get an extra resuscitating tube and keep it in your car. No ambulance ever arrives at the scene of an auto accident in time to restore a non-breathing patient; somebody else on the scene will have to do it. You? Why not? It might be someone in your own car.

Carbon monoxide exhaust from an internal combustion engine may strip the transport of oxygen from lung to brain. Hemoglobin, the red pigment in the blood cells, under normal conditions forms a loose combination with oxygen in the lungs. The blood then goes to the brain or other body tissues where oxygen is easily exchanged for carbon dioxide. The body cells use the oxygen, and the carbon dioxide is carried back to the lungs and exhaled. The loose combination that hemoglobin makes with oxygen in the lungs, and carbon dioxide in the tissues, makes a handy exchangeable chemical system.

Carbon monoxide, on the other hand, makes a tight combination with hemoglobin that prevents oxygen pickup in the lungs and exchange for carbon dioxide in the tissues. Anoxia (lack of oxygen) leads to unconsciousness; the individual may be breathing but her tissues are not getting oxygen. Her location—near the fumes of an internal combustion engine with inadequate ventilation—should tell you what the trouble is. And she will be bright cherry red color, resulting from the combination of carbon monoxide and hemoglobin. Time is essential. She must be gotten away from the fumes by one who can hold his or her breath long enough. Scuba-diving gear, if nearby, can be used to rescue such a person. If she is breathing, watch her closely; if she stops, assist her. She will have an awful headache when she does come around.

This, of course, will never happen on your boat because you will always check the venting of your engine room. Even on a sailboat, this is an absolute must.

Nature is kinder to the person who bleeds than to the one in respiratory arrest or interference. Compensatory mechanisms go to work at once that can sustain life for a considerable period of time in spite of severe bleeding. Injury to body tissue—skin, muscle, bone, or viscera—causes a host of chemical reactions in the body. The blood cells and platelets sludge (clump together) and markedly speed up clotting of the blood when it gets to the site of injury.

The blood pressure drops rapidly, too; blood loss is minimized and clots form readily under less pressure. Arteries in the extremities and outlying part of the body constrict so that the remaining blood goes around a shorter circuit through the head, brain, lungs, and other vital organs. The heart beats faster, which also helps.

This vasoconstriction of the arteries may entirely close down a vessel in an arm or leg wound. I do not suggest that you allow nature to stop major bleeding unassisted. Do the things we have talked about earlier in this chapter, and do them promptly. But in assessing a critical situation, remember that an injured person who is both bleeding and apneic dies of lack of oxygen rather than shortage of blood. Emphasis is necessary because bleeding is dramatic and attracts attention, whereas apnea is rather passive.

The need for sterile surgical gloves in "first aid" may be questioned. However, there is no doubt that after one scrubs his or her hands before caring for a wound requiring extensive care, suturing, or performing an operation, the additional use of sterile gloves is preferred. In a very urgent emergency, sterile gloves can be immediately used, thereby cutting down the risk of infection. There are many other times–during a rectal exam, for example–when you will be glad you stocked sterile gloves for your trip.

CARDIAC ARREST AND CARDIOPULMONARY RESUSCITATION

A less likely but more complicated situation than the case presented at the beginning of chapter 1 arises when both breathing and circulation (heartbeat) are arrested. Two common causes are near drowning and heart attack.

Either situation presents a victim who

1. is unconscious and unresponsive,
2. makes no breathing movements,
3. has no pulse or heartbeat (see figure 3),
4. makes no voluntary movements,
5. has extremities cold to touch, lips often blue in color.

Management:

1. Start mouth-to-mouth breathing as described on pages 3–5.
2. After giving two breaths, begin external cardiac compression (cardiac massage), using the following procedures for adults. (See figure 7 for child compression.)
3. Locate the sternum (breastbone) by following the curve of the ribs to the midline (see figures 4 and 5).
4. Place the heel of your right hand firmly over the middle of the sternum, making sure it is not over the abdomen (which is below the rib cage). Have fingers parallel to the ribs.
5. Place your left hand firmly on top of your right hand (see figure 6.)
6. Lock the thumb of your left hand around your right wrist to prevent slipping when pressure is applied.

There is no need to take the pulse for a whole minute. It should be sufficient to take it for 10 seconds and multiply the result by 6.

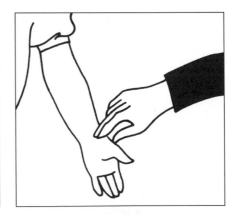

The heart beats about 90 to 110 times each minute in a young child and about 80 to 100 times in an older child. Each heartbeat forces blood around the arteries of the body and can be felt as a pressure wave over several points of the body.

The WRIST is the commonest place to feel the pulse. Gently press the tips of your index and middle fingers over the under side of the wrist at the base of the thumb.

7. Apply pressure vertically down from the shoulder, keeping your left elbow straight and using body weight as a compressing force.
8. Continue cardiac compression and mouth-to-mouth in the ratio of fifteen cardiac compressions to two breaths mouth-to-mouth —five sets to the minute.
9. Continue until the patient revives, begins to breath on his own, and the heartbeat can be felt on the chest or the pulse at the wrist.

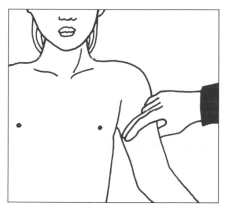

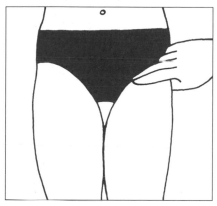

ARM: Hold the upper arm as shown in the diagram and gently press your index and middle fingers against the arm bone.

GROIN: Gently press your index and middle fingers over the middle of the groin fold.

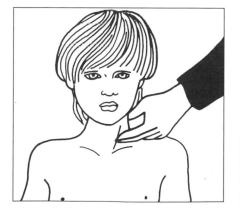

NECK: Place your thumb around the back of the child's neck and place your index or middle finger on the side of the neck next to the windpipe and gently press towards your thumb.

Fig. 3. A child's pulse is apt to be more difficult to feel than an adult's. The locations are the same for both but the adult rate at rest is seventy to eighty times per minute. Sketches modified from *First Aid Fast and Simple,* by Dr. James Witchall, published by Bay Books Pty., Ltd., Kensington, New South Wales, Australia.

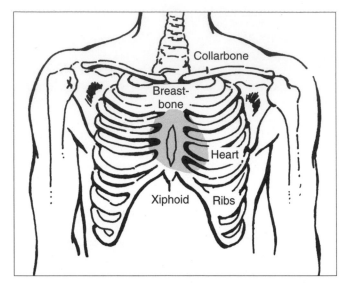

Fig. 4. Anatomy of external cardiac compression. Modified from *The Surf Life Saving Manual,* published by the Australian Life Saving Association.

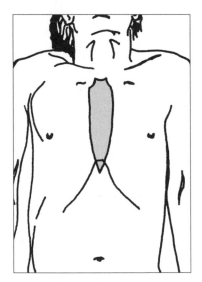

Fig. 5. Location of the compression points.

In most regions an ambulance service, the Red Cross, or other first-aid training organization will give courses in CPR and have a mannequin upon which to practice. *Never practice external cardiac compression on another person.* Everyone, sailor or landlubber, should learn this technique. It can save a life because, as has been said earlier, the

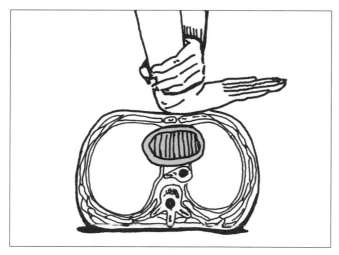

Fig. 6. External cardiac compression.

need for its use is always immediate—within seconds to one minute of the cessation of breathing and heartbeat from whatever cause. It would be advisable to have two persons trained in CPR onboard your vessel, and they should be capable of performing two-person CPR.

NEAR DROWNING

A victim of submersion needs instant action at his present location. Six minutes' submersion is usually fatal, but longer survivals have been recorded.

1. Start mouth-to-mouth resuscitation wherever the victim is located. Continue until he is breathing on his own. Continue during any necessary movement of the victim to a more suitable location.
2. Watch the victim carefully for twenty-four hours longer. Be prepared to assist breathing whenever necessary.
3. If possible, keep the patient's head low—the first sign of recovery if he is unconscious may be a violent spasm of the diaphragm that jets a huge quantity of water and stomach contents out his mouth. If his head is upright he may inhale this with his first breath which will likely be fatal. If his head can't be kept low, watch carefully for this and cover his nose and mouth briefly.
4. If there is no recovery continue resuscitation mouth-to-mouth for a least an hour.

5. If the water was dirty, give Keflex in full dosage (to prevent pneumonia) and Doxycycline (to prevent gastroenteritis) for five days. Before giving antibiotics, try to determine whether an allergy exists.

Prognosis (What to Expect) in Near Drowning
If the victim is conscious, choking, and spluttering, he will probably recover. If he is unconscious but has a good heartbeat and pulse (don't let a search for this interfere with your mouth-to-mouth efforts), he will more than likely recover. Some spluttering and/or voluntary movements after twenty minutes is a good sign recovery is on the way.

If the victim is unconscious and pulseless, with no heartbeat, the situation is doubtful for recovery, but such sufferers have been saved. If there are enough crew about to maintain breathing support and cardiac massage, there is always a chance and it is worth the effort.

Discussion—Near Drowning
If the submersion victim has breathed water into the lungs (10 percent do inhale water) this changes the mechanics of lung function and makes it hard for normal breathing to be restored.

Salt water is hypertonic and causes a stiffening of the alveoli (air sacs) so many of them collapse and do not fill easily with air when breathing resumes.

Fresh water is hypotonic in relation to blood and so excess water is absorbed into the blood flowing through the capillaries (small blood vessels) of the lung. This dilutes the blood and diminishes its capacity to carry oxygen.

Depth of Compression

Patient	Compression Site	Method	Depth
Adult	Lower half of sternum	2 Hands	40–50 mm (1.5–2 inches)
Child to 8 years	Middle of sternum	1 Hand	25 mm (1 inch)
Baby & infant to 1 year	Middle of sternum	2 Fingers	15 mm (½ inch)

Fig. 7. Note the ratio of compressions to breaths differs for children and infants. For children, the ratio is 5 to 1 at a rate of eighty to one hundred compressions per minute. For infants under one, the ratio is the same, but the rate should be one hundred per minute.

It is for these reasons that once normal breathing starts the sufferer must be watched carefully for twenty-four hours by someone able to resume mouth-to-mouth assistance at a moment's notice.

Prevention of Near Drowning
Adult sailors need no particular advice other than to wear life jackets at appropriate times, and always when alone on deck especially after dark. Or they may elect to wear safety harnesses at such times. A safety line is mandatory in rough weather and when on deck after dark, and can easily be installed by running a stout line from backstay to forestay through the center of the vessel. Crew people can clamp their safety harnesses onto this wherever their location.

It is worth noting that the majority of sailors go overboard when the weather is mild. When seas are heavy almost everyone remembers to move slowly and hang on.

See chapter 19 for measures to prevent near drowning in children.

HYPOTHERMIA

Immersion in extremely cold (20°C, 68°F) water may produce hypothermia, a reduction of the core temperature of the body. This diminishes oxygen need and may enable longer survival of immersion. A number of years ago a small boy was frozen in the ice in Lake Michigan for several hours and survived without brain damage.

It can be difficult when a person (child or adult) has been immersed in extremely cold water to determine if he or she is alive or dead. The victim will be cold to touch, unconscious, pulseless, apneic, pupils dilated—to all appearances dead. If the rectal temperature is 94° (core temperature is likely lower but the standard clinical thermometer registers no lower) and the patient is warmed passively with blankets and cardiopulmonary resuscitation until rectal temperature rises to 96°F, he or she may be one of the very lucky survivors who fall into the hands of someone who recognized the condition and knew how to treat it.

PENETRATING CHEST WOUNDS

Penetrating chest wounds, those that make a hole through the chest wall into the pleural spaces around the lungs, are dangerous. The lungs hang in two vacuum sacs—the pleural cavities. A person breathes by expanding the chest wall to which these sacs are attached. The pressure of the outside air forces air down into the lungs. A hole in the chest wall destroys the vacuum (see figure 8), and though the chest wall expands, the air pressure is then equal on both the inside and outside of the lung, and the lung does not fill.

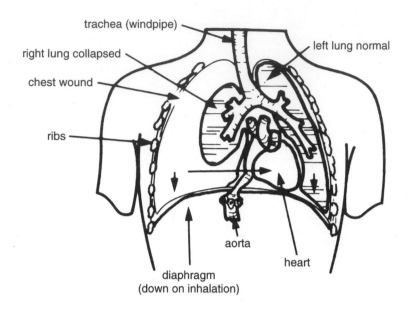

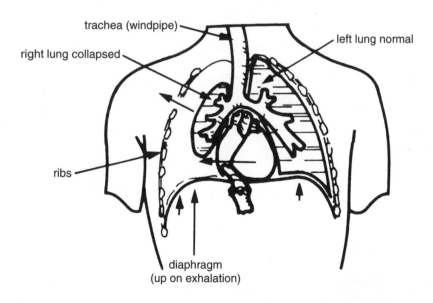

Fig. 8. *Top,* Inhaling—open chest wound. Note air entering chest through wound and not going into right lung; left lung normal. *Bottom,* Exhaling—open chest wound. Air passes out through chest wound; right lung has not filled with air.

You can help this by mouth-to-mouth breathing. And you had better close the hole in the chest wall as soon as possible; put some type of dressing in or on it to seal it off. The air already in the pleural sac will be absorbed slowly once the hole is closed, and the lung will presently begin to work again.

PAIN CONTROL

Illness or injury alerts the brain that all is not well with the body. Once you have found the cause of the pain, you should take measures to reduce or eliminate it. In cases of injury, changes in position or immobilization of the affected part, such as in a fractured leg, are very important. Giving reassurance and handling the casualty firmly and calmly cannot be stressed enough. This will immediately instill confidence in you, and frequently this feeling reduces the victim's perception of the degree of his or her disability, thereby reducing the perception of pain.

The analgesics or "pain killers" that you carry aboard all have advantages, disadvantages, and dangers. As always, you must consult the package inserts to understand more about these important medicines. For mild to moderate pain, use the following guidelines for dosages:

1. aspirin, 300 mg tablets, give two every four hours.
2. Tylenol Extra Strength, 500 mg, give two every four to six hours.

For moderate to severe pain, use Tylenol with codeine (Tylenol #3) and give one or two tablets or capsules every four to six hours.

For severe pain, use Demerol, 100 mg, by deep intramuscular injection, every three to four hours. This controls pain in most cases. One can decrease the amount of Demerol needed by concomitantly giving Phenergan, 25 mg, also by deep intramuscular injection. This gives a sedative effect and also decreases nausea. A good dose to start with would be Demerol 75 mg with Phenergan 25 mg. It is suggested that Phenergan not be used more frequently than every eight hours (careful review of the package insert is very important). The patient must be carefully monitored, and you should tend toward smaller doses. Remember, if your crew member has a significant decrease in respiratory rate or is less responsive, do *not* give further analgesics at that time.

Avoid all narcotics in the following situations:

1. with a person who has abdominal pain, at least until the illness or injury has been assessed;
2. with an unconscious patient;
3. with a person who has a history of unconsciousness for any period following previous head injury;
4. with a person who has hypothermia.

Discussion

At the beginning of this chapter we indicated that lifesaving first aid was simple enough. But now, having saved a life at some distance from medical aid, you are going to have to deal with problems that are not quite so simple. Fortunately you will have time to consider your actions. Depending upon the availability of medical help, you are going to have to be a doctor for a varying period. The remainder of this book is directed toward helping you decide what you can and cannot do until such aid is available and how to do it.

A word of warning—this book will not make you a doctor; use a real doctor when one is available. Above all, do not apply what I am about to discuss with you in a foreign port where there are doctors who may not understand your language; you may think them inferior to the doctor you remember back home, but you are in their country and they must take care of you and your crew under their own laws. Doctors everywhere are striving to treat people, even strangers, to the best of their ability. You must trust them when they are available. Treat only your own crew members and only when organized medical care is unavailable to you.

One sad example should suffice. A well-trained thoracic (chest) surgeon was on a fishing trip in a foreign port. At the end of the day's fishing, a member of another boat's crew had a cardiac arrest on the pier. This surgeon applied his skill and restored the man's heartbeat. However, the patient died a few hours later in a hospital. The surgeon was charged with manslaughter. He had no license to practice medicine in the country where this occurred. He was freed finally, but only after a long and disagreeable experience.

I repeat—at sea, with your own crew and no help available, do all you can, as we shall try to help you do it. Even though physicians are greatly concerned about professional liability today, many states have Good Samaritan laws to protect those who responsibly provide, without any fee-for-service charge, treatment in an emergency situation. However, turn the patient over to others better qualified—even though they may not seem so to you—as soon as possible.

CHAPTER 2

Fractures, Sprains, and Dislocations

You engage in a tacking duel with your nearest competitor from San Pedro Harbor Light to Point Fermin. Wind is westerly, 18 knots; you carry the 180 percent Genoa and make short tacks to stay out of the channel current that drives to leeward.

You come about onto the starboard tack headed out to sea; there is a yell from a winch tender. His right hand is crushed between the Genoa sheet and the Barient drum. You luff up to free his hand; he falls to the deck, pale and hurt. The right hand, which he holds in his left, is turning blue and swelling massively; the fourth and fifth fingers are cocked off at peculiar angles. The skin is not broken.

1. Control pain with analgesics (see page 17).
2. Gently straighten out the bent fingers. (See below #2 for severe pain.)
3. Apply a well-padded universal arm splint with fingers in position of function (see section on splints below and figure 9).
4. Elevate the splinted extremity in a sling or hooked onto the overhead of the bunk.
5. Leave fingertips exposed; loosen bandage when necessary and reapply.

Crush injuries of the hand and wrist occur frequently on sailboats and can damage extremely important structures.

The five steps outlined are basic treatment for all simple fractures (those that do not have an open wound extending to the broken bone).

It is wise to get this patient to a hospital as soon as possible. Treatment of severe crush injuries of the hand, with or without fractures, demands sophisticated equipment and knowledge.

If you are far out to sea and unable to get to port:

1. Continue the splint and elevation.
2. Medicate to control pain. Demerol 100 mg by intramuscular injection may be needed if pain is severe, at three- to four-hour

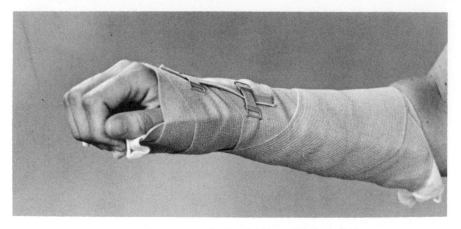

Fig. 9. Universal arm splint applied; fingers in position of function.

intervals. The dose of a narcotic should vary according to the age of the patient and the severity of the pain. The stated dose is average for a 150-pound person. Older people and young people should have lower doses.

3. Coldness and tingling or lack of feeling in an extremity that is splinted are causes of concern. The circulatory status and swelling *must* be checked daily. For untoward symptoms or excessive swelling, the splint must be loosened to relieve the tightness.

4. After twenty-one days, remove the splint and gently move the uninjured fingers. This will reduce the swelling somewhat in the rest of the hand.

5. Replace the splint but leave the uninjured fingers unbound so they may move.

6. Over the course of the next two weeks, gradually increase the motion of the hand and fingers.

7. When movement no longer hurts, remove the splint.

8. *Always* see an orthopedic surgeon when back in port.

Do not worry about whether there is a fracture. This treatment is equally effective for crush injury without broken bones.

SPLINTS

Simple fractures (broken bones with overlying skin intact) are treated by immobilization in a splint until the broken bone ends heal together. A splint is a simple device long enough and strong enough to immobilize the broken bone, one joint above and one joint below the fracture. It must be well padded to protect the skin and bony parts from pressure sores. Splint-padding material or cast liner is not expensive and does not require much storage space (see figure 10). If you lack a supply of cast liner, materials such as strips of cloth, towels, etc., make a good substitute.

The best splints for use on shipboard are the cardboard type which stow flat and are folded up for use. Two or three of these lengths suitable for the arms and legs of your crew members, plus the universal hand splint, will serve your needs for a cruise of any length.

Pneumatic splints also stow flat, and after being applied to the fractured extremity, are inflated (see figure 11). It is *important* to do this only with mouth pressure, otherwise *it may stop circulation.* Never keep a pneumatic splint on for more than twenty-four hours due to possible vascular or nerve damage from constriction.

Traction splints are also available and are popular with ambulance services, but these require more stowage space and are difficult to apply correctly. The traction is an advantage but the hazards on shipboard outweigh the advantages, in my opinion.

If you lack prefabricated splints, many materials aboard may be employed. Use your imagination: Swab handles, winch handles, heavy pillows, sail battens, or navigational charts folded to the requisite stiffness can be used satisfactorily.

I once saw an excellent splint fashioned from four segments of a broom handle that enabled a camper to bring his wife comfortably 400 miles out of the desert to the hospital. He was a certified public accountant by trade but proudly designed and created this splint for his wife's broken knee.

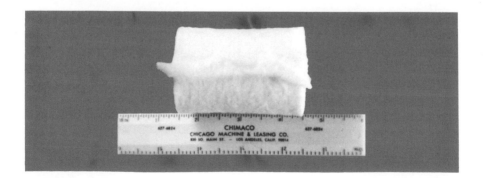

Fig. 10. Cast liner.

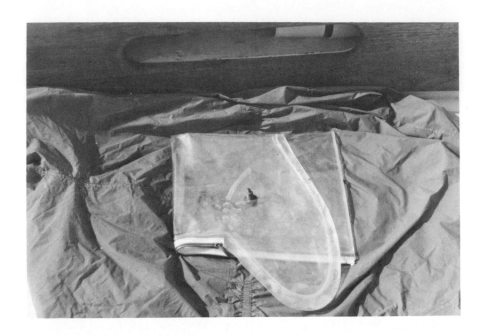

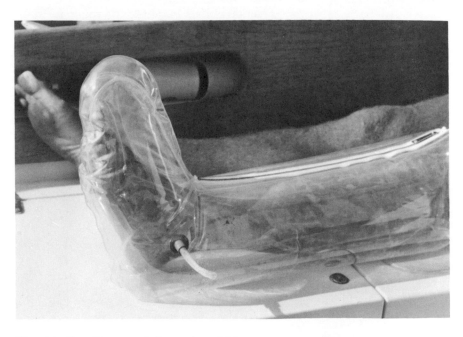

Fig. 11. *Top,* Pneumatic leg splint folded for storage. *Bottom,* Pneumatic leg splint applied.

SIMPLE FRACTURES

A member of your crew steps into an open hatch, falls forward, and catches his left mid-leg on the hatch coaming. There is a loud crack; he lands on the deck with his leg angled awkwardly and exquisitely painful. He cannot stand on it; the effort is agonizing. The skin is unbroken.

1. Examine the leg gently; cut away his trousers to get a good look at it.
2. Feel his shin. You will probably find the edges of the broken bone.
3. Let him lie unless he has fallen into an inaccessible position. If he has, wrap the broken leg firmly to the uninjured one with an Ace bandage before you move him to a convenient spot to work on him.
4. Give him Demerol 100 mg by injection (see figure 12).
5. Clean the overlying skin well with Betadine, then inject approximately 20 cc of 1% Xylocaine into the fracture site.
6. Straighten out the right, unbroken leg with the ankle held to a right angle.
7. Sight through the right great toe to the center of the right knee-cap. This is the normal weight-bearing line.
8. Brace yourself; take a firm grip fore and aft on the left ankle.
9. Have assistant hold the injured man under the armpits.
10. Pull the broken leg slowly out straight; this is traction. Be steady; watch the broken part. Do not force the bone ends to poke out through the skin—this would compound the fracture.
11. Slowly bring the broken leg into the proper weight-bearing line.
12. Traction should make the injured leg feel better.
13. Your assistant pulls from above; this is countertraction.
14. You feel the bones move into an end-on-end position. Keep the traction on and slowly lift the leg. Let a second helper slide a folded-up and padded cardboard splint into place. This must be long enough to go from toes to well above the knee and fit snugly.
15. The second helper should first wrap the leg and splint firmly together with an Ace bandage. Leave the toes exposed.
16. Now very slowly let off the traction (your pull) and countertraction (your first helper's pull under the armpits).
17. Two of you carry him to his bunk. Detail another person to manage the splinted leg. Coordinate your movements.
18. Elevate the splinted leg.
19. Continue pain control with Demerol, as needed. If you use Demerol or Tylenol #3 for a few days, you may have to give a laxative because these drugs are constipating.

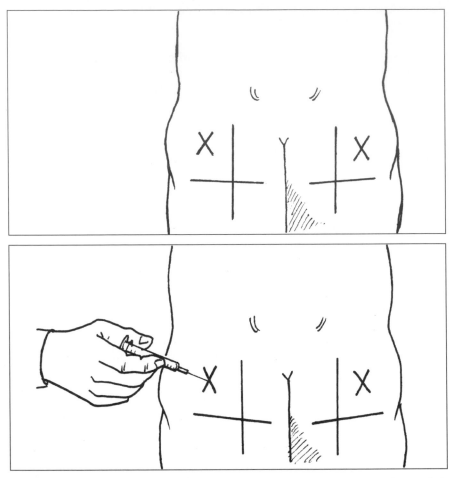

Fig. 12. *Top,* Area for intramuscular (IM) injection—upper outer quadrant of either buttock. *Bottom,* Angle of needle insertion. Whenever possible, have the patient stand up straight when receiving a deep intramuscular injection in the buttocks. In this position the injection causes less discomfort.

20. Watch his toes. If they become very swollen, blue, numb, and at the same time, painful, the splint is too tight.
21. Reapply the traction and countertraction.
22. Unwrap the bandage around the splint, including the final turn. Hold traction; wait for toes to "come alive" and feel warm.
23. Rewrap the splint, then let off the traction.
24. Do this as often as necessary; the broken leg will hurt at the site of the fracture. This is different from the pain of a splint that is too tight.

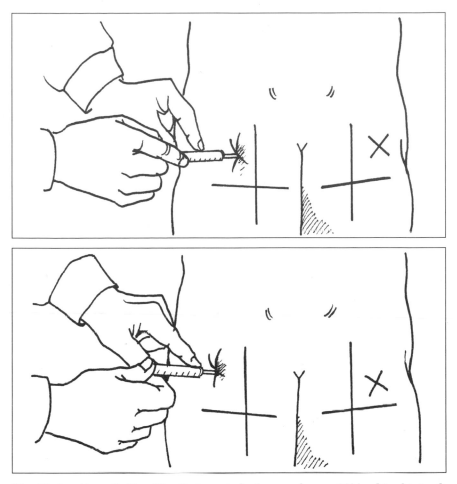

Fig. 12. (continued). *Top,* Needle inserted, plunger drawn. If blood is obtained, move the needle—it is in a vein. *Bottom,* Injection completed.

25. You will want to get outside help; this fracture requires a minimum of three months to heal. Meanwhile, maintain splint, control pain, and watch the circulation in the toes.

SIMPLE FRACTURES OF OTHER EXTREMITIES

Manage fractures of the elbow and shoulder differently. The location of important nerves and blood vessels close to these bones makes it imperative that minimum efforts be undertaken to line up or reduce the

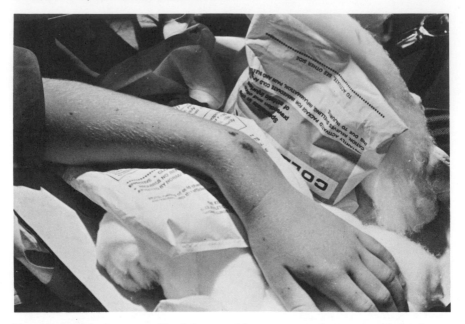

Fig. 13. Simple fracture of both bones of forearm; angulation at mid-third.

fracture. Such injuries should be gently straightened out so you will not drive a broken bone end through an artery or nerve.

Fractures of the forearm (between the elbow and wrist) often produce a striking deformity (see figure 13). It is safe to straighten these enough to apply a splint handily, but watch the bone ends. Never compound a fracture by pushing the ends through the skin. Be gentle; apply steady nonjerking traction.

The hand splint is useful for forearm fractures. After the splint is applied, the limb can be brought to a right angle at the elbow and held in a sling around the neck. Then, additional support can be offered from elbow to upper arm. Wrap a firm, wide bandage around the chest, over the elbow and arm.

Fractures of the arm (shoulder to elbow) are usually not remarkably deformed. They present a problem for splinting because it is difficult to immobilize the joint above (the shoulder).

It is best to splint an arm fracture with the elbow at a right angle. A sling will help and if immobilization is still inadequate as noted by severe, increasing pain at the fracture site, the arm and forearm may be bound to the chest wall. Usually, this is not necessary.

Fractures of the ankle are splinted without traction. If severe deformity is present, gentle molding to the appearance of the normal side will help.

As in all fractures, rough, irregular movements are forbidden. If there is a question in your mind, it is better to splint the broken bone in the position in which you find it. You will thus do no further harm. This is a prime principle of all medical practice.

SPINAL FRACTURES

Dr. Arthur Davis, a fine orthopedic surgeon and racing sailor, devised the modern method of reducing broken backs. He cut a ring life buoy in half and fastened the two halves together to make a rounded splint over which he stretched the patient's broken back. This extension brought the cracked vertebrae back into line and a cast was then applied. This principle is still used, although the equipment has been changed.

The danger from spinal fractures is injury to the spinal cord, resulting in paralysis. Such damage may occur at the time of accident. In this case, not much can be done about it. It may occur following improper handling after the spine is broken. This is a preventable tragedy.

Acute forward bending (flexion) causes most spinal fractures. Cervical spine fractures commonly occur as a result of diving in shallow water; the head strikes the bottom and the full weight of the body bends it forward.

This type of injury and extreme tenderness over the neck bones on the gentlest feeling (under no circumstances allow the patient's head to bend forward when you examine him) would cause you to suspect a neck (cervical) fracture. There is rarely any apparent angulation of a broken neck. Minimal movement laterally will cause pain at the site of the broken vertebra.

If the patient is paralyzed (cannot move his feet or hands), the spinal cord is damaged. Care for him as described in chapter 8, "The Unconscious Patient."

If you suspect a cervical fracture and there is no paralysis:

1. Do not move the patient.
2. Sit above him, with his head between your legs.
3. Put one hand on either side of his jaw; pull gently but firmly up without bending his head forward.
4. Now have someone else give him an injection of Demerol (75–100 mg) if he is in pain.
5. Hold traction and have your assistant slide a board under his neck and upper back. Any rigid structure that will immobilize the entire spinal column will suffice. This will lessen the risk of damage to the spinal cord, which is the main objective in this case.

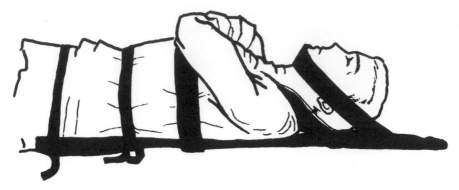

Fig. 14. Suitable splint for fractured spine.

6. If the board is narrow, wrap a bandage about his head to hold his neck firmly in place (see figure 14). If the board is wider, pad either side of his head out to the bandage.
7. Slowly release traction.
8. Have two or three persons lift him so his trunk and the splint remain level.
9. Carry him level to his bunk and put him there, board and all.
10. Keep him flat and splinted until you get to help. Keep him that way as long as possible.
11. Control pain with continuing medication.
12. Urinary retention with subsequent need for a catheter may occur.
13. Abdominal distension may be seen on a reflex basis.

Should a diving accident occur and the patient still be in the water, it would not be possible to exert traction on his neck. Swim alongside him and bend his head backward, gently (extension). Then float a board under his neck and back and fasten him to it firmly before you bring him out of the water.

But wait a minute! Did you check his breathing? Did he need to be resuscitated? Remember, this comes first.

Fractures of the lower (thoracic and lumbar) spine are rare injuries on shipboard. These are also caused by forceful flexion. Management is similar—rigid splinting before movement and control of pain. Traction for these injuries is rarely possible on shipboard.

BROKEN NOSES

Broken noses are not serious unless they bleed too much, too long. All broken noses bleed, but most of them stop within an hour or so.

1. Clean your hands and put on surgical gloves. Apply pressure. Pinch the nostrils together with a hot *(not cold)* rag, or just your fingers.
2. If this does not work, take the forceps from the first aid kit and pack some cotton into the bleeding nostril.
3. If bleeding continues and the patient is alarmed, Tylenol #3 will often quiet him and aid in stopping bleeding. Valium 5 mg might also be given to relax the patient.

If all these measures fail and bleeding is continuing at a profuse rate, you will have to make a nasal pack:

4. If the Tylenol #3 has not decreased the pain sufficiently, supplement with Demerol 75 mg.
5. Get the Foley catheter in its prepackaged envelope (see figure 15).
6. Fill the little balloon with 4 cc of air to test it; then deflate it.
7. Decide which nostril is bleeding.
8. Sit your patient up with firm support behind his head.
9. Lubricate the Foley catheter with a surgical lubricant, Vaseline, or in a desperate situation, even salad oil.
10. Pass the catheter into the bleeding nostril; it will encounter resistance, but press firmly and gently on.

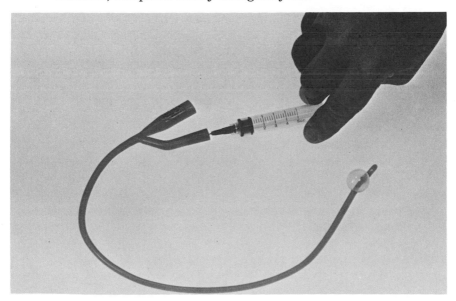

Fig. 15. Foley (in-lying) catheter; air-injection method of testing balloon before insertion.

11. Sudden end to the resistance tells you the tip of the catheter has passed into the nasopharynx (chamber behind the nose).
12. Inflate the balloon in the Foley catheter with the amount of air recommended on the package. If the patient is too uncomfortable decrease the volume of air in the Foley balloon.
13. Pull the catheter forward firmly; the balloon will close off the back side of the nasal chamber. All of the bleeding should be coming out of the front of the nose. If there is any blood running down behind (ask the patient), pull the catheter forward more vigorously.
14. Anchor the catheter firmly to the patient's forehead with several strips of adhesive. The pressure will be uncomfortable; if it is not, you do not have it tight enough.
15. Pack nostril in front of catheter balloon with sterile gauze lubricated with Vaseline.

You now have the nasal chamber packed fore and aft and bleeding will be limited to that small space.

You may need to give Demerol freely (100 or even 150 mg every three hours) because this pack is misery. Add Valium 5 mg (a tranquilizer) by injection every four to six hours if your broken-beaked crewman cannot tolerate the pack with Demerol alone; add Phenergan 25 mg, which produces a synergistic effect with Demerol, to give greater pain relief without having to increase the dose of Demerol. Check the patient carefully to be sure his or her breathing has not been depressed by the Demerol and Valium before adding Phenergan.

16. In twelve hours, remove the gauze from the nostril; if blood flows, repack the nostril and do not disturb the catheter. (But, if blood is running down the throat behind, trim it a bit tighter to the forehead.)
17. Check every twelve hours. If there is no bleeding when the gauze is removed from the nostril, wait four hours.
18. When you are sure bleeding has stopped, deflate the balloon of the catheter and very slowly and gently draw it out.

A final word of warning: Do not be in a hurry to remove the catheter. It is difficult to replace.

OTHER COMMON FRACTURES

Fractures of the Clavicle
Fractures of the clavicle (collarbone) are often caused by a sideways fall onto the shoulder. They cause immediate local pain and tender-

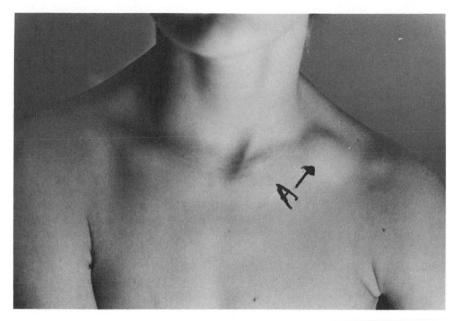

Fig. 16. Fracture of mid-third left clavicle (collarbone); tender swelling at A.

ness. The injured individual cannot raise his arm beyond 90° from his side without severe pain.

Feel the uninjured clavicle and then the suspicious one. Run your fingers along from the breastbone to the shoulder. Seek irregularity, swelling, tenderness, or even jagged bone ends beneath the skin (see figure 16).

Reduce a fractured clavicle in the following manner:

1. Clean your hands and put on surgical gloves. Give Demerol 75–100 mg by injection.
2. Seat the patient on a stool and stand directly behind him.
3. Clean the skin well with Betadine and inject local anesthesia (about 10 cc of 1% Xylocaine) into the fracture site.
4. Have one assistant on each side raise each arm as high and as far backward as possible.
5. The operator grasps the top of each shoulder from the back to front; put your right knee between the patient's shoulder blades. Pull hard.
6. When reduction is accomplished as determined by the movements of the bones and possibly an audible snap, fashion a heavy figure-eight bandage running under both armpits across the back of the neck (see figure 17). In front, pass over the bony prominences of the shoulder, not under the armpit.

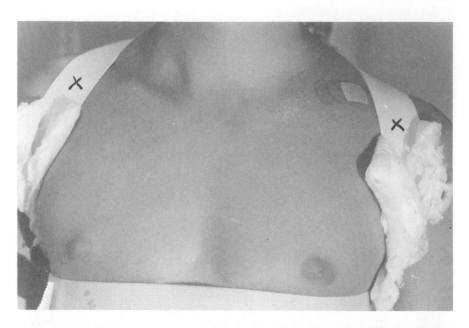

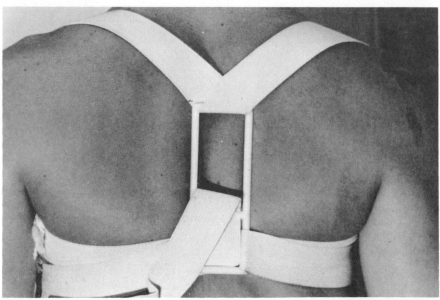

Fig. 17. *Top,* Front view, clavicular splint; note pressure is on bony points of shoulder, at X's. (Band-Aid covers site of local anesthesia injection.) *Bottom,* Rear view, clavicular splint; same pressure can be held with a heavy figure-eight bandage.

7. When the reduction and splinting are accomplished, if an arm becomes numb or begins to swell a great deal, release the bandage; it is cutting off the axillary artery to the arm. A fractured clavicle, even if unreduced, will heal. Do not risk loss of blood flow to the arm.
8. If the reduction is unsuccessful or if the patient cannot tolerate the figure-eight bandage as described, put the arm in a sling. Be sure the sling holds the wrist to the chest wall, thereby limiting external rotation of the arm which would be harmful to a clavicular fracture.

Fractures of the Pelvis

Pelvic fractures are often caused by severe crush injuries. A sailor who gets caught between dock and boat or who has heavy gear fall across the pelvis can suffer such an injury.

Pressure on the lateral sides of the pelvis over the two iliac crests and/or pressure from front to back from the pubic region to the lower lumbar region, which causes sharp pain in a localized area, suggests a pelvic fracture.

The treatment for such fractures is rest in bed and Demerol or Tylenol #3 (see page 17) when needed, for pain.

One complication which may occur in a severe pelvic fracture that can be helped on shipboard is interference with urination. Swelling around a broken pelvic bone near the bladder may obstruct urine flow.

If the patient with suspected pelvic fracture is unable to void for a period of eight to ten hours, it will be necessary to pass a catheter (see chapter 6 for technique). Leave it in-lying and start Bactrim DS (double strength), one tablet every twelve hours, with a glass of water at each dose, as long as the catheter is in place. As with any antibiotic or sulfa drug, one should check for any known drug allergy.

Fractures of the Wrist

The Colles' fracture (named after the seventeenth-century Dublin surgeon) occurs at the wrist. It is caused by a fall on the outstretched hand (see figure 18). Pain and inability to move the wrist accompany it.

Though it is difficult to maintain this fracture after reduction, it will do little harm to attempt the following:

1. Clean your hands and put on surgical gloves. Administer Demerol 75–100 mg by intramuscular injection.
2. After cleansing overlying skin well with Betadine, inject 10 cc of 1% Xylocaine into the fracture site.

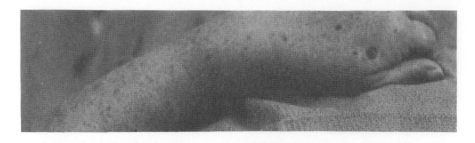

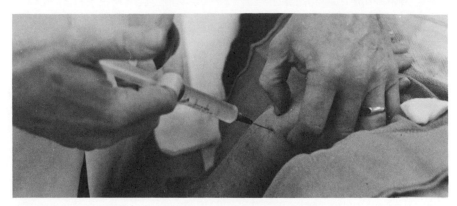

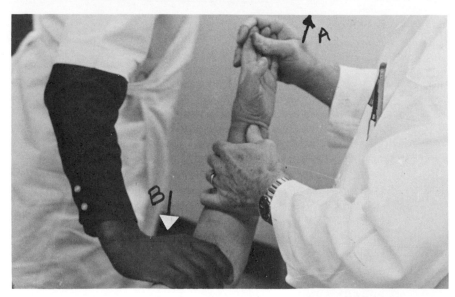

Fig. 18. *Top,* Broken wrist (Colles' fracture). *Center,* Injection of local anesthesia into fracture site. *Bottom,* Traction (A) and countertraction (B) for reduction of broken wrist.

34

3. Have an assistant apply counteraction to the arm just above the elbow (see figure 18).
4. Hold the patient's hand in your opposite hand (patient's left to your right, or vice versa).
5. Exert steady, firm, straight traction while your assistant maintains steady countertraction. Do not jerk but do not be afraid to pull.
6. When bones move at the fracture site, cock the hand up sharply, put your thumbs across lower ends of broken bones and slide them down into place. Straighten out the wrist.
7. Reduction will be accompanied by movement of bones at the fracture site and often a grating sound or click.
8. Hold the wrist until a universal arm splint is strapped firmly to the wrist and hand.
9. Administer follow-up care as for other fractures.

Fractures of the Toe
Fractured toes usually occur with a stubbed toe—a barefoot sailor, a deck cleat, a dark night. They are not fatal but may be very painful. Splint by taping them firmly to adjoining toes. The patient should wear a shoe until bare-foot walking is painless.

SPRAINS

Thumbs, fingers, and ankles are frequently sprained; wrists and necks less often at sea. A thumb bent too far backward stretches or tears the ligaments that support the joint. Often a small fracture accompanies it.

If such an injury to the thumb or finger is accompanied by great pain and huge swelling that is aggravated by any attempt to move the part, treat it as a fracture. Give medication for pain (Demerol or Tylenol #3) and apply the universal arm or other splint (with the fingers in the position of function). Keep the splint in place, loosening it when necessary, for three weeks. It is safe enough to remove the splint for a trial of motion after two weeks. If this is successful, it suggests a mild sprain and the splint may safely be removed. If pain persists, then the splint must be reapplied.

A sprained ankle without accompanying fracture need not put its owner out of action. You can find out in this way (see figure 19):

1. Seat the injured person with the calf of his leg resting on a support, injured foot and ankle sticking beyond.
2. Shave his ankle and leg to mid-calf.
3. Paint his foot, ankle, and leg to mid-calf with compound tincture of benzoin.

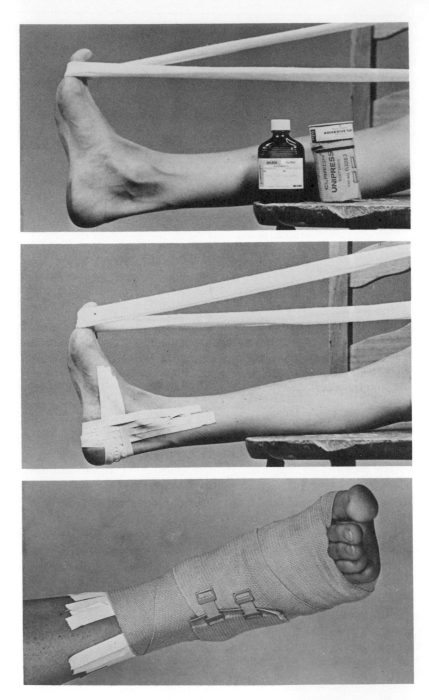

Fig. 19. *Top,* Position and supplies for ankle strapping (therapeutic test for possible fracture). *Center,* Alternate anchors and stirrups. *Bottom,* Completed bandage, ready for test of weight bearing.

4. Run a light sheet around his great toe. Have the patient hold both ends and maintain the ankle at a 90° angle.
5. Cut a strip of 1-inch adhesive tape long enough to reach from six inches above the ankle inside his leg, under the foot, and up to the same level on the outside of the leg. This is a stirrup.
6. Mold the stirrup smoothly down the inside of the ankle (after the compound applied is dry and sticky). Run it smoothly under the foot to the outside of the leg; pull up and stick it down.
7. Cut another strip of 1-inch tape long enough to reach from the base of the great toe, around the ankle horizontally and to the base of the fifth toe. This is an anchor.
8. Alternate anchors and stirrups until the ankle is covered.
9. When the weave is finished, wrap an Ace bandage over the tape firmly.
10. The smoother the tape, the more comfortable the bandage.
11. Now have the patient stand up on his good foot and put weight gradually on the taped ankle.
12. If he can begin to walk about with slight discomfort, he has a mild sprain. Take him off the sick list but send him to light duty.
13. If weight bearing hurts a lot, he has a bad sprain with torn ligaments and/or a fracture. Put an ankle splint over the adhesive strapping and consign him to his bunk for three weeks or until the end of the cruise, whichever comes first.
14. If he can walk at first, but over the course of twelve hours the pain becomes more severe, do the same as step 13.

You have just completed a therapeutic test. You lose no time because the boot will splint the ankle so he can walk on it.

This dressing was devised by a British Army surgeon to keep soldiers with sprained ankles active. It will do this for sailors, too. Note that no tape passes around the ankle. If it swells, loosen the overlying Ace bandage and reapply.

In an extreme situation radiotelephone contact with an orthopedic surgeon could provide advice as to whether a local anesthetic injection into the joint is advisable.

DISLOCATIONS

The dislocation of finger joints is one of the commonest you will see. The diagnosis is obvious, but you cannot tell whether there is a fracture as well.

Get to a finger dislocation within a few moments. It will be numb for a bit. A straight pull pops it back painlessly. (Remove all finger rings at once; cut off the ring if necessary). After you relocate a dislocated finger, apply a splint in the position of function (for one finger). Leave it on for fourteen days at least, to allow the strained joint ligaments to heal.

Another common dislocation is the shoulder. After a twisting force, you will note:

1. An immobilized, painful arm held tight to the body.
2. Severe pain throughout the whole shoulder area.
3. A depression over the shoulder joint as compared to the normal one on the other side.

You may safely reduce this as follows:

1. Give Demerol 100 mg by injection.
2. Allow forty minutes for the patient to relax, reclining on a bunk in any comfortable position.
3. Turn the patient onto his or her abdomen. Place the good arm under the forehead and let the dislocated shoulder hang out over the edge of the bunk.
4. Apply traction steadily on the arm down towards the deck.
5. Increase pull gradually. If you aggravate the pain, the muscles will tighten down and defeat your attempted reduction.
6. Be in no hurry. If you get tired of pulling, have the victim hold 5–10 pounds in his or her hand (a bucket of water, etc.).
7. It will reduce "all at once," usually with an audible snap.
8. The relief from pain will be great.
9. Apply a sling and bandage the arm to the side of the chest with elbow at a right angle.
10. Keep it splinted for three weeks. Then gradually begin motion.
11. Have the patient bend forward with the injured shoulder and arm falling free, and swing the hand in ever-widening circles. Start gradually and extend this as fast as possible daily until the full range of shoulder motion returns (circumduction exercises).

CHAPTER 3

Compound Fractures, Wounds, and Amputations

COMPOUND FRACTURES

A sudden squall hits the *Sea Witch* at 0400 hours on a Monday halfway between Tarawa and Penrhyn in the Gilbert Islands. Before you lower the mizzen staysail, it pulls a pad eye from the deck. The deck watch ducks and throws up a hand. It takes the full force of the flying block.

The sailor falls to the deck aft the cockpit, his left hand torn and bleeding. Bone ends poke through the skin. He sits up, inspects his ruined hand, unbelieving.

1. Wrap his hand firmly in a suitable splint (cardboard or other) on the spot (see figure 9).
2. Assist him to his bunk.
3. Give him 100 mg of Demerol by injection.
4. Prepare the following: Three quarts of water boiled twenty minutes and cooled with the cover on, Betadine, elastic bandages, gauze squares.
5. Scrub your hands five minutes at galley sink with Betadine and fresh water. Rinse with part of the sterile water. Put on surgical gloves.
6. Remove the splint you applied in step 1, then press gauze squares firmly over wound with left hand (see figure 20).
7. Scrub the skin around the wound with Betadine and sterile water. Hold the gauze in your right hand. Have an assistant pour sterile water onto the gauze and the wound as needed.
8. Shave the area around the wound.
9. Now remove the gauze in the left hand from the wound. Throw it away. Inject 10–15 cc of 1% Xylocaine into the cleaned wound surfaces.
10. Take fresh gauze and more Betadine. Scrub inside the wound, including the broken bone ends, thoroughly. Get it clean; remove chips of loose bone and dirt. Leave bone fragments that are attached.

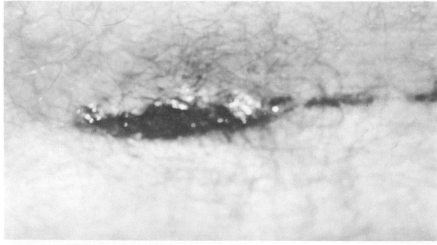

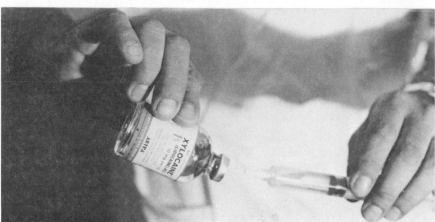

Fig. 20. *Top,* Deep leg wound. *Bottom,* Drawing local anesthesia from multiple-dose vial. Cleanse rubber stopper with alcohol wipe before puncture. *Opposite top,* Injection of local anesthesia to numb wound. *Opposite center,* Scrub-out of wound. Afterward, it may be closed or packed open. *Opposite bottom,* Wound packed with sterile gauze.

11. Rinse three times with sterile water.
12. Press fresh dry gauze onto the wound until bleeding from the wash-up stops (four to ten minutes).
13. Observe the patient's right uninjured hand; mold the broken bones of the left hand into a similar configuration.
14. Squeeze a generous dollop of an antibiotic ointment into the wound.

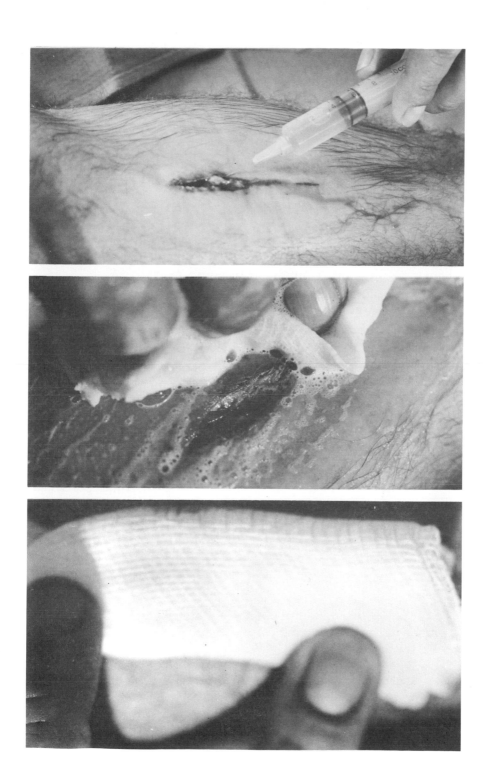

15. Place sterile gauze over the whole wound.
16. Apply an Ace or other bandage firmly over the gauze.
17. Apply a universal hand splint with the fingers in the position of function (see figure 9) and secure it with a second firm bandage.
18. Elevate the splintered arm above the patient's head.
19. Give Keflex 500 mg, four times daily, *or* Cipro 500 mg tablets two times daily for one week.

This completes the primary definitive treatment of a compound fracture. This case involves the wrist but the treatment applies to any compound fracture. Should a leg be involved, after the wash-up and dressing and before you splint the extremity, it is advisable to reduce the broken bone ends to an end-on-end position by traction and counter-traction. See description for simple fractures in chapter 2.

Follow-up Care
Follow-up care of the compound fracture:

1. Maintain the splinted position.
2. Control the pain with injections of Demerol 75–100 mg every four hours as necessary. An oral analgesic should be substituted when applicable.
3. Prevent infection as stated in #19 above.
4. Change the wound dressing as often as necessary, i.e., when soaked with blood and serum, preferably before it begins to smell. This interval may be hours, days, or (in cool climates) several days. As with all re-dressing of open wounds, scrub your hands and put on surgical gloves.
5. Observe the patient's fingertips every four hours for coldness and numbness; loosen the bandages if the splint becomes too tight. Remember to loosen both bandages.

To change the dressing, follow this procedure:

1. Prepare sterile water: twenty-minute boil and cool with lid on.
2. Give Demerol 100 mg by injection if patient has had none for the past three hours.
3. Remove and discard the dirty dressings.
4. Wash the skin and the wound gently with Betadine and sterile water. Remove all crusted serum and exudate.
5. Rinse the wound gently.
6. Cover with triple antibiotic ointment.
7. Apply clean gauze and a bandage over the wound.

8. It is better to wrap wound bandage outside the one holding the splint to the part. Then you may expose the wound without loosening the splint. This maintains reduction.
9. You have to care for the patient, too. A broken leg ties him to his bunk for the rest of the cruise. He may hobble painfully to the head with help but a bottle and pail are simpler. A bedpan is a handy item. You may lug one thousands of miles and never use it but if you have space, take one along.
10. Tylenol #3 and Demerol are constipating drugs. Give a good laxative such as a Dulcolax suppository if your patient goes several days without a bowel movement or he may develop a fecal impaction which he cannot pass. It will have to be dug out by hand.
11. Narcotic drugs plus inactivity and pain may make urination difficult. Force fluids and encourage him to void before his bladder becomes distended and too uncomfortable. Often a man will be able to void if he can touch the deck with just one foot.

If he becomes too distended (twelve to eighteen hours without urinating), you may have to catheterize him (see chapter 6). Do not be in a hurry to do this. He will void spontaneously before he ruptures his bladder, although the agony of waiting may be more than you and he can bear.

Discussion of Fractures
Basic treatment for all fractures is:

1. Immediate reduction of the part to normal alignment. If the patient is in an inaccessible spot, bind the broken limb firmly to a sound one, then move him to a better location.
2. Splint the broken bone ends plus one joint above and one joint below, when anatomically possible.
3. Maintain immobilization until healing is complete.
4. If the fracture is compound, splint in the deformed position first, cleanse the wound to prevent bone infection, then remove the first splint. Reduce the fracture and reapply the splint. Leave the skin wound open.

It has been known for centuries that immediately following a fracture the tissues are in a state of local "shock." Pain is nil. This period only lasts a few minutes. Shortly pain begins and nearby muscles set into spasm, which locks the broken bone ends wherever they lie.

There is considerable bleeding, too, at the fracture site from the marrow cavities of the broken bones and from injury to the surrounding soft parts. A hematoma (blood clot) develops. Swelling and further stiffening and immobilization of the tissue follow.

Reduction will be more likely to succeed if it is done while the part is numb and before spasm and swelling develop. After reduction, spasm helps to hold the reduction. Firm, steady pull on any fractured extremity that draws it into a normal position like the opposite uninjured limb should do no harm.

Make an exception for a compound fracture. If reduced before wash-up, the bone ends carry dirt into the wound. Be swift with a compound fracture. You may finish the wash-up before the numb period ends. If not, you can surely wash up and splint in an hour; the swelling usually does not appear for two hours or sometimes longer.

Local anesthesia, 30 cc of 1% Xylocaine injected into the fracture site under aseptic precautions, will relieve pain and help in the wash-up and reduction. Note that more than 30 cc of Xylocaine injected at one time may be toxic.

It is a working rule among surgeons that there is no timetable for healing of fractures. This is determined by X-ray examination at regular intervals. So, lacking X rays, you will need to maintain the splint on a major bone fracture until help arrives. A broken leg, for example, may require from three to five months or even longer to heal completely.

Fractures heal by spanning the gap between broken bone ends with an interlacing network of fine fibrils derived from the local hematoma. Delicate cells (fibroblasts) creep out along this network to form soft scar tissue. A second type of cell (osteoblasts) deposits calcium that hardens the scar into callus. It is this solid callus that welds the bone ends firmly together. The whole process takes several weeks or months. Such tissue growth is easily interrupted by movement of bone ends that tear the latticework of fibrils much as a spider's web is torn by movement of anchoring bushes.

Infection at the fracture site replaces the tissue growth with a different type of activity—one aimed at destroying the invading bacteria. Healing is impeded by infection. The infection must be eliminated either through surgical drainage or through the action of an antibiotic or by both.

Strict immobilization and absence of infection promote prompt healing of any fracture. If, on the other hand, the healing process is delayed by undue mobility or infection, subsequent repair becomes prolonged and difficult. Bone grafts and other surgical operations are often needed.

If you can prevent infection and maintain immobilization of a fracture on shipboard, you will save your shipmate a good deal of suffering and disability when the doctors take over.

WOUNDS

Wounds, like the charms of Shakespeare's Cleopatra, are of infinite variety. Size, location, cause, and hazard to life and limb may vary. A knife cut on the finger is a wound; so is a leg ripped off by a shark's teeth. The latter at first glance seems more serious but sailors have survived shark bite while other sailors have died from apparently simple lacerations.

The basic treatment of wounds is:

1. Stop major bleeding.
2. Clean your hands, put on surgical gloves, and wash up the wound.
3. The wound must be closed within six hours to prevent the infection that most certainly would follow in the coming hours. Suturing muscle should not be done without the advice of a physician. Make no attempt to close tendons, nerves, or other deep-lying structures. (These can be repaired secondarily by the appropriate surgical specialist where one can anticipate a far better result.)
4. Bandage.
5. Change bandage as necessary.
6. Remove sutures (stitches) when wound is healed.
7. If infection develops, remove all skin closure (Steri-strips, staples, or sutures). Spread the wound widely.
8. Apply moist warm compresses to the infected wound.
9. Give systemic antibiotics when indicated. See "Follow-Up Care of Closed Wounds" on page 49.

To close a wound with Steri-strips:

1. After wash-up (as for compound fractures) and control of bleeding, dry wound edges thoroughly.
2. Paint both edges of wound with compound tincture of benzoin.
3. When it is dry, stick a Steri-strip firmly to one skin margin. Pull the wound together and stick strip to opposite skin edge (see figure 21).
4. Repeat until the wound is well covered with Steri-strips.
5. You may substitute adhesive tape butterflies, store-bought or homemade.
6. Bandage firmly over Steri-strips.

To suture (sew up) a wound, assemble:

1. Prepackaged silk or nylon 2-0 or 3-0 sutures attached to curved cutting needles.
2. Sterile prepackaged needle holder.
3. Scissors.

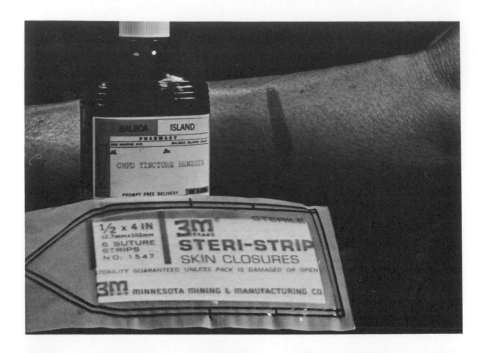

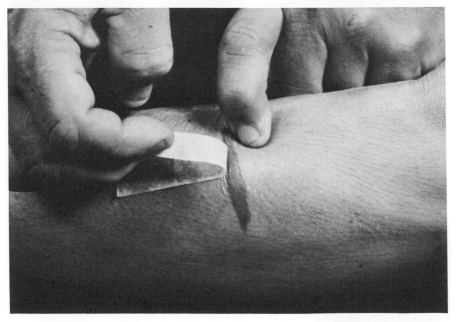

Fig. 21. *Top,* Steri-strip materials and, *bottom,* technique.

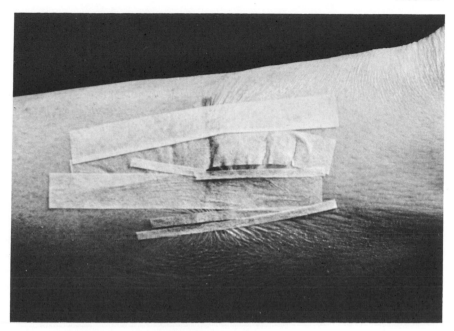

Fig. 21 *(continued)*. Completed Steri-strip closure.

4. Toothed tissue forceps.
5. Sterile, prepackaged 4" × 4" gauze squares.
6. 10 cc hypodermic syringe and sterile prepackaged No. 21 or No. 22 needle.
7. 1% Xylocaine without epinephrine.

This is ideal. If your first aid kit is incomplete, substitute:

1. Sail or other sewing kit for sutures.
2. Pliers for needle holder.
3. Razor blade or knife for scissors to cut sutures (thread).
4. Clean cloths, 4" × 4", for sterile gauze squares.
5. There is no satisfactory substitute for hypodermic needles or Xylocaine (see figure 22).
6. If you are unable to inject local anesthesia, sew without it. Tylenol #3 by mouth or intramuscular Demerol will make the process bearable for the victim.

All unsterile (i.e., not prepackaged) instruments and supplies can be sterilized by boiling for twenty minutes in a covered pan.

To sterilize previously opened prepackaged plastic syringes or instruments, soak in alcohol for one hour; do not heat—heat melts the plastic.

47

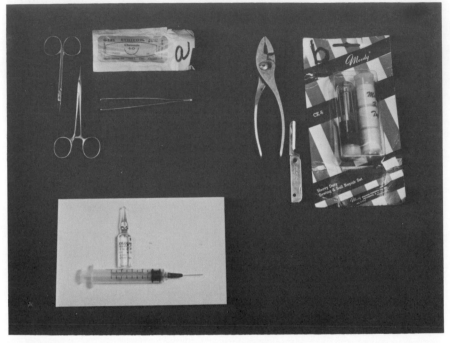

Fig. 22. *Top left,* Surgical sewing kit. *Top right,* Available substitutes. *Bottom left,* No substitutes for syringe and local anesthesia.

Details of wound suture:

1. Wash up and put on surgical gloves, as described in compound fracture.
2. Inject wound edges with local anesthesia as shown in figure 24.
3. Do not inject more than 30 cc of 1% Xylocaine without epinephrine in an adult. Review the package insert for the proper dose for a child and when repeated injections are needed.
4. Apply constant pressure over gauze to stop bleeding caused by the wash-up and injection of local anesthesia (four to ten minutes).
5. Check anesthesia; touch sensation remains, but pain is eliminated.
6. Place gauze squares, unfolded, about the wound to make a sterile field.
7. Open the suture; put the needle in the needle holder (see figure 23A).
8. Grasp one wound margin (side of cut) near the end with tissue forceps. Turn it up to 90° angle. Push the needle through, perpendicular to the skin edge (see figure 23B).

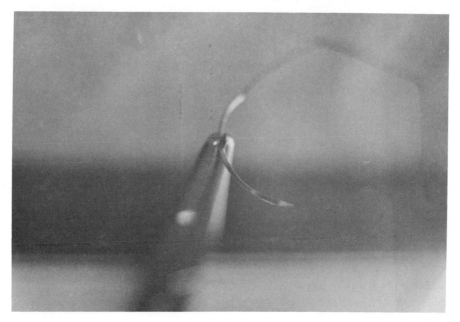

Fig. 23A. Placement of needle in needle holder; suture is attached.

9. Grasp the opposite wound margin and repeat step 8.
10. Knot the bitter end of the suture to the standing part to close one end of the wound.
11. Repeat steps 8 and 9. Fashion a running stitch that closes the whole wound. Keep sides even.
12. Tie a second knot at the other end.
13. Cut the suture free and discard (see figure 23C).
14. Apply antibiotic ointment to the suture line. Bandage firmly.

The procedure is the same whether you use the materials described or have made substitutes.

Wound Staples
An alternative technique to close lacerations is by the use of staples. Following step #6 above, use the WECK Visistat stapler. It is a disposable unit with simple directions included for using up to 35 staples—which should be ample even for extensive trauma on a single patient.

FOLLOW-UP CARE OF CLOSED WOUNDS

The procedure is the same for Steri-strips, butterflies, stapled, or suture-closed wounds.

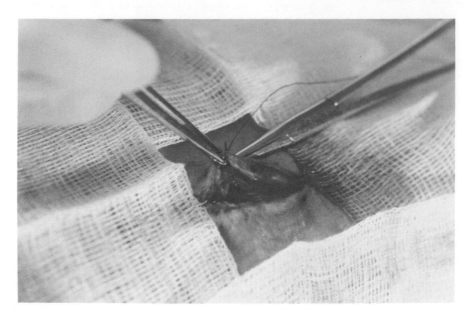

Fig. 23B. First stitch of wound suture. Note wound margin turned up to a right angle.

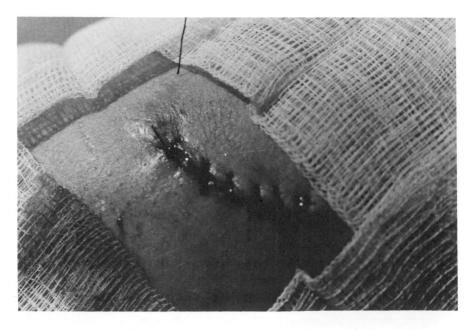

Fig. 23C. Completed suture line; suture cut away.

1. Change the outer dressings only if they get wet or very dirty. Then scrub your hands and put on surgical gloves.
2. Remove all dressings in five to seven days; the wound should be healed. Removal of sutures, staples, Steri-strips, etc. is usually done after five days. On lower extremities or areas subject to a lot of motion, it's probably best to wait seven days. Try taking out every other closure; if the wound tends to open, leave the other closures in. As always, don't hesitate to use your communication equipment to get a physician's advice.
   a. Pull Steri-strips or butterflies off wound edges gently with the pressure in the longitudinal direction of the wound (otherwise the wound may be pulled open again), or
   b. Cut sutures at each turn and remove the several fragments.
   c. Follow the directions that come in the sterile package with the WECK staple remover.
3. Suspect infection at any time after closure if there is:
   a. Increasing pain in the wound after twenty-four hours.
   b. Swelling about the wound.
   c. Bulging of the wound.
   d. Pus dripping from the closure.
   e. Increasing redness and heat about the wound.
4. If the wound appears infected:
   a. Remove the dressings.
   b. Remove all Steri-strips or sutures.
   c. Spread the wound wide open.
   d. Place gauze pads into and over the wound, moisten with salt solution (1 tsp table salt to 1 qt fresh boiled water).
   e. Keep the part at rest and elevated.
5. Suspect wound infection plus sepsis (blood poisoning) if the patient has:
   a. Chills and fever (temperature above 101°F).
   b. Red streaks out from the wound.
   c. Swollen tender lymph nodes at the groin or armpits.
   d. Step 3, points a–e.
6. Wound infection plus blood poisoning (sepsis) calls for:
   a. Bunk rest for the patient.
   b. Broad-spectrum antibiotics: Cipro 500 mg two times daily.
   c. All procedures under step 4.
   d. If infection appears to progress, add Metronidazole 250 mg three times a day.
7. Stop wet-dressing the wound when local infection subsides as shown by:
   a. Less pain and swelling.

      b. Pus stops forming.

      c. The base of the wound becomes pink and healthy.

8. Stop systemic antibiotics when the patient's temperature is normal for twenty-four hours and the wound shows foregoing changes.

9. After infection subsides, leave the wound open to heal in from the bottom. Never close it. Dress as needed with antibiotic ointment and dry gauze. If the cosmetic result is poor, it can be corrected ashore.

DISCUSSION—SOFT-PART WOUND HEALING

Soft-part wounds heal much like fractures except that the end product is scar tissue instead of bony callus. Fine fibrils extruded from a blood clot crisscross the wound. Young fibroblast cells creep out along these miniature suspension cables to bridge the gap. They mature into firm scar tissue in eighteen to twenty-one days.

Infection and/or excessive motion of wound surfaces interrupt proper healing. The wound treatment aims to prevent both. The outside scrub removes bacteria from the surrounding skin so washing the wound and suturing will not carry them into the wound itself. It resembles the skin preparation done before any operation. Gauze pressed into the wound protects it from splash during the scrub. The wound cleansing removes dirt, bacteria, and dead tissue that encourage infection.

Careful hemostasis (stopping bleeding) after cleansing minimizes blood clot in the closed wound. Some clot is needed for healing but an excess promotes infection. Antibiotic ointment over the wound closure checks bacterial invasion until serum seals the wound shut.

Wound closure shortens healing time by narrowing the valley that healing cells must fill. It also restricts movement of wound edges that might otherwise shear off the delicate developing tissue bridges.

All wounds are contaminated because bacteria are ubiquitous. The bacteria in a fresh wound, however, lie quiet for some hours like newly planted seeds in a field until warmth and moisture incite growth. Usually the body defenses will destroy them before this happens. If not, the bacteria begin to grow and reproduce.

Infection turns the formerly peaceful healing process into a holocaust of battle. Millions of white blood cell shock troops swarm into the combat along widely dilated arterial pathways. Some of these cells wall in the infection while others gulp down (phagocytose) the deadly bacteria in suicidal attacks. The body count of dead cells and bacteria in the center grows steadily. Small wonder that trampled nerve ends cause pain, that the part swells, and that the heat of violent struggle can be seen and felt though the overlying skin.

Should this first line of defense conquer the infection, there remains a wall of living leucocytes (white blood cells) around the dead cells in the center. This is an abscess and the center is pus. Pus under pressure can strangle living cells and rally the invader to a renewed attack. Avoid this danger by opening the wound wide to relieve pus pressure. Encourage continued drainage by wet dressings until you see no more pus.

Should the infection overcome this first line of defense it will progress as red streaks in lymph vessels radiating out from the wound. Lymph nodes in armpits or groin will swell and hurt. If it reaches the bloodstream, sepsis (blood poisoning) causes chills, high fever, and severe illness. Systemic antibiotic treatment is necessary to conquer this invasion. The proper use of such drugs is described in chapter 7.

Leave a wound open once drained, lest you trap some infected material and renew the infection. Such an open wound will heal by secondary intention. This takes longer and makes more scar than a wound that heals by first intention (i.e., without infection), but it will heal.

Most clean wounds on shipboard should be closed. The less gaposis, the less scar necessary to heal it, and subsequent repair of tendons or nerves will be easier. You may do harm if you attempt to repair deep structures. Close only the skin.

OPEN WOUNDS

Avulsed wounds, those with the skin torn away, will not close. Approximate wound edges where possible and pack the remaining area with sterile gauze plus antibiotic ointment. Change this when wet or soiled. A wet dressing, warmed by body heat, is an ideal culture medium for bacteria.

Badly mangled wounds or those with ground-in dirt (see figure 24) are best packed open. A good general rule is: If there is any question about closing a wound, pack it open. You will get a bigger scar but will be more likely to have an uninfected wound.

Puncture Wounds

Puncture wounds—deep, narrow holes such as a nail would make—require special treatment. Tetanus (lockjaw) bacilli and gas gangrene bacteria are obligate anaerobes (they can grow only in the absence of oxygen).

Anaerobic conditions develop at the bottom of a deep puncture wound if the top seals over before the bottom heals.

To treat a puncture wound:

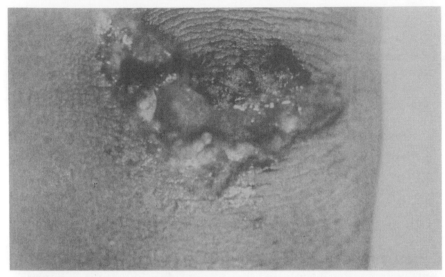

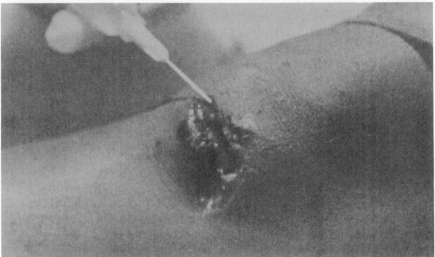

Fig. 24. *Top,* Mangled knee wound with dirt ground into dead tissues. *Bottom,* Injection of local anesthesia before wound scrub-up.

1. Thorough wound cleaning is your main concern. Cleaning an open wound is best accomplished by washing with copious amounts of water and scrubbing or washing as much as possible with Betadine or even hand soap and water.

   Should you feel that this attempt to clean the wound was unsatisfactory, and gently probing produces no result, then proceed to step #2.

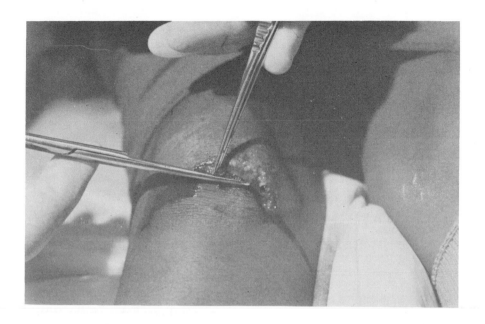

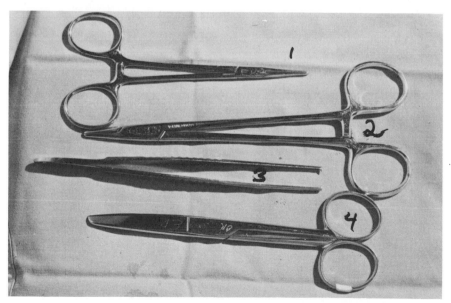

Fig. 24 (continued). Top, Cutting away dead tissues and ground-in dirt with a scissors. The wound will be packed open. Bottom, Instrument kit for wound excision and/or suture: (1) hemostat, (2) needle holder, (3) tissue forceps, (4) scissors. Sterilize by boiling for twenty minutes.

2. Inject local anesthesia (1% Xylocaine) into and around such a puncture wound, core it out, pack it open with antibiotic ointment on sterile gauze to heal from the bottom up.

All crew members, prior to going to sea, should have received a primary immunization course of three doses of tetanus toxoid vaccine—and had booster injections of 0.5 ml every ten years. Individuals who have completed primary immunization and who sustain wounds which are minor and uncontaminated should only receive a booster dose of tetanus-toxoid preparation if they have received none within the preceding ten years. For more serious and contaminated wounds, it is appropriate to give a booster if the booster was not given within the last five years. If the details of the primary immunization are questionable, an immediate booster dose is in order. Treat the patient with Keflex 500 mg, four times a day.

CRUSH INJURIES

These injuries are characterized by massive swelling with skin and soft tissue bruising. There may be concomitant loss of skin. If the circulation of the blood to the part is affected, then the problem will be further compounded.

A "compartment syndrome" may occur when the pressure within the limb is increased to such an extent that irreversible tissue damage occurs.

The proper management, once the condition is recognized, is to treat by relieving the pressure surgically. Before proceeding with opening the fibrous tissue layer that encases the muscles, nerves, and blood vessels (fasciotomy), it would be highly desirable to receive instructions by radio from a general surgeon or orthopedic specialist.

TRAUMATIC AMPUTATIONS

These may result from tearing or cleavage. Your immediate concern is to stop bleeding from the stump. The severed part is likely not to be viable, but it may be possible for a doctor to reattach it if surgery is not delayed for too many hours. The best approach would be to keep the severed part cool. Wrap it in a sterile dressing and place in a plastic bag. The bag should then be placed in a second plastic bag containing ice chips. Do *not* place the part directly into the ice and do not allow it to freeze.

Radiotelephone communications should also immediately be instituted to secure an emergency surgical opinion. Even in distant waters there have been occasions when Search and Rescue units have gotten desperate cases to sophisticated medical care in a short time. Don't fail to give your crewmember every chance. You'll never know if he or she could have been helped if you don't consider this an ultra-emergency.

AMPUTATIONS

You are not likely to be unlucky enough in your cruising to encounter a white whale that mangles the leg of one of your crew. But it is possible you may have to amputate an arm or leg.

Before undertaking such a major surgical procedure you must realize that serious complications must be prepared for, and death is a distinct possibility. The immediate problem is to control hemorrhage with tourniquets and pressure, and pain with injectable narcotics. Don't try to make the decision yourself. Use your communication equipment and if your setup is adequate it is rare that you cannot reach emergency help and talk with a surgeon. There may be alternatives and "watchful waiting" may be the way to go. *If* you must proceed, try to do it with the surgeon assisting by radio. It could make all the difference in the outcome, and it is only fair to your patient and crewmember to do so.

Remember, amputate only to save life. It is a terrifying experience for both the skipper and the injured crewperson. Save any extremity—however badly mangled—that has essentially normal color (i.e., not dead white or dusky) and that bleeds from exposed vessels within the area of injury or beyond. Splint it carefully; control pain with Demerol 75–100 mg by injection every three to four hours as needed. Prevent infection by giving Cipro 500 mg three times daily until clean healing progresses. This may be a week, two weeks, or even longer. Meanwhile, make every effort to secure help.

In spite of such care the injured part may die and severe spreading infection may begin. The patient will suffer chills, high fever (oral temperature to 104° F or even higher), or perhaps delirium. Pain in the injured extremity can become progressively worse and worse. The dead tissue will turn black or dusky and stink. Red streaks may climb up the extremity; lymph nodes in the groin or armpit will swell up and hurt (see figure 25).

Gangrene may also develop when bleeding in an extremity thwarts control for several days. Each time you loosen the tourniquet or pressure bandage, vigorous bleeding gushes from the wound. Shortly, either the patient bleeds to death or the extremity becomes gangrenous because the continued pressure cuts off adequate blood flow.

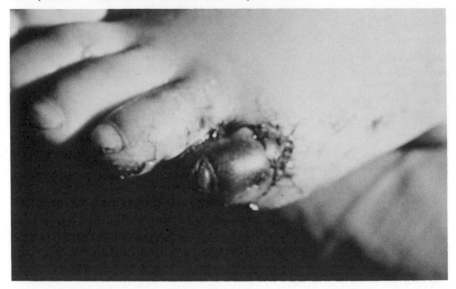

Fig. 25. Gangrenous fifth toe, seven days post-suture. Dark area is anesthetic; surrounding foot is red, swollen, and tender. The toe will be amputated and the wound packed open. Healing time is approximately two weeks.

If you have a plentiful supply of ice aboard, you may delay amputation of a gangrenous extremity for some hours or days, perhaps long enough to reach port. Proceed thusly:

1. Give Demerol 100 mg by injection if none has been given in the past two hours.
2. Place a tourniquet tightly around the limb two inches above any dead tissue or pus. Once placed, never remove it.
3. Pack the limb below the tourniquet in ice. Keep replenishing the ice.

Within twenty-four hours the pain lessens, the temperature and pulse drop towards normal (less than 100°F and less than 100 beats/ minute), and the patient is obviously better. You may safely continue the treatment until the temperature and pulse rise sharply and remain elevated. Do not panic at moderate daily fluctuations of temperature and pulse. The sustained progressive rise of either demands intervention. Amputate only when you are sure in your own mind the patient is going to die if you do not.

You are the skipper and will have to be the surgeon. Anyone can amputate a finger or toe. Simply inject 10–15 cc of 1% Xylocaine into the base and cut it off. Use a sterilized pair of heavy shears or a heavy knife. Control bleeding with a tourniquet of rubber bands or fine ties. Control pain with Demerol and dress the wound afterwards as often as necessary. Leave the wound open.

If a foot and leg below the knee are involved you can likely amputate successfully. Above the knee you may elect to leave the outcome to fate, for amputation at this level is difficult and much more hazardous.

The major danger of the operation is bleeding. It may occur at the time of amputation if the main vessels are not controlled or it may occur up to a week after the operation if infection loosens a blood clot in a major vessel.

If you decide you have the courage to go ahead, here is what to do:

1. Get the ship on the steadiest course possible.
2. Select a firm bench or table to which the patient can be lashed and which provides access on all sides.
3. Pick two assistants who do not faint at the sight of blood.
4. Log the date, time, and ship's location. Write that in your opinion the patient's life is in danger unless the amputation is carried out. You are not a doctor but feel competent to remove this offending part and thus save his or her life. Have the patient sign and both assistants witness this. Such a consent has no legal standing. However, it is a generally accepted principle of law that what one does in an effort to save a life is usually acceptable.

You will need the following supplies:

1. 1% Xylocaine without epinephrine,
2. A 20-cc sterile syringe with a 3-inch needle, size 18 or 20,
3. A sharp knife with at least a 3-inch (and preferably a 6-inch) blade,
4. Three or four hemostatic forceps,
5. Three dozen sterile gauze squares. If these are not available, tear toweling or sheets into 4" × 4" squares and sterilize by boiling for twenty minutes. Then allow to cool and dry before use.
6. Two stout rubber or elastic tourniquets. Mooring slack holders or heavy shock cord are suitable as are nylon or manila line (¼").
7. A bucket,
8. Six 2-0 silk sutures. If you have no prepared sutures, substitute fishing line, stout packing string, or sail sewing cord and needles (sterilize by boiling twenty minutes).
9. A hacksaw or other type of saw. Sterilize by wiping it several times with antiseptic solution, especially the teeth. A hacksaw is particularly good. Soak the blades in a pan with rubbing alcohol or any other antiseptic for a couple of hours prior to the operation. Have several blades.

10. A roll of adhesive tape, 2" × 10 yards,
11. Two Ace bandages, 2–3",
12. A single-action pulley and some means of fastening it to the lower end of the bunk or onto the overhead,
13. Demerol, 50 mg/ml, 1-ounce bottle,
14. Hypodermic syringes and needles
15. Scissors, sterilized.

Now you must prepare the patient:

1. Give the patient 125 mg of Demerol plus 10 mg of Valium by separate injections one hour before the operation.
2. Also administer Rocephin 2 grams deep intramuscularly 30 minutes to one hour before surgery.
3. Shave the entire extremity above the infected area.
4. Scrub your hands and put on gloves. Then scrub the entire leg from groin to toes ten minutes; use fresh water and Betadine. Make all strokes from clean to dirty area, downward.
5. Lash the patient firmly to the operating table on a sheet or blanket.
6. Place the bucket immediately below the operative site.
7. Assign a second assistant to monitor the tourniquet.
8. Stand on the right side of the patient if it is the right leg or on the left side if it is the left leg.
9. Have your first assistant stand directly across from you.
10. Lay your sterile instruments on a clean towel on a handy stand.
11. Scrub your hands for ten minutes with Betadine and a brush or a soap scrub pad. Rinse with sterile water. Put on surgical gloves.

Now for the details:

1. Scratch a circle around the leg at the level selected for amputation, two inches above any dead tissue, pus, or infection. Use knife tip or a needle.
2. Draw 20 cc of Xylocaine into syringe; inject it into the scratched circle just under the skin. It should bulge the skin all the way around the circle.
3. Refill the syringe and inject around again at a deeper level. Refill the syringe and repeat until you have injected 75–100 cc of Xylocaine and have completely infiltrated tissues from skin to bone in a circle all around the leg. This is a dose that may be toxic and even cause convulsions, but it is a life or death situation so you must be prepared for this possibility. Valium, preferably given intravenously, may be needed for convulsions.

4. Wait five minutes. Test the anesthesia with a pin below your injection circle. Wait until the leg is numb both on the surface and deep before you begin to operate. The sense of touch may persist but when pain is gone, anesthesia is satisfactory.

5. The second assistant should tighten the tourniquet firmly about the lower thigh. As you operate, if there is any persistent bleeding, tighten the tourniquet until it stops. This is essential; the tourniquet must be tightened until bleeding is controlled. Have a spare tourniquet handy.

6. You have selected a site for amputation at least 2 inches above any infection or pus or dead tissue.

7. Take your knife, cut clear around the leg through the skin and fat. Follow the scratch. The skin is tough and white; the fat is yellow. Allow a moment for the skin to retract. Fascia glistens white; red muscle is below. Then as high as possible towards the retracted skin, cut the muscles all the way around. These will jump and twitch away from your knife but make it as straight as you can. Your first assistant wipes the wound dry of blood with gauze squares so you can see to cut.

8. Continue circular incisions clear around the leg each time until both bones are exposed. There are two bones in the leg: the tibia (large) and the fibula (small).

9. Use the knife to scrape the bone clear for an inch of all muscle attachments and membrane.

10. Inject some local anesthesia (10 cc of Xylocaine) into the periosteum, the tough membrane stuck fast to the bone.

11. Unfold a gauze square, wrap it around the divided skin and muscles. Have your second assistant pull up on this hard while your first assistant holds the leg in a handy position.

12. Saw through both bones of the leg. Bones are hard, so brace yourself and the leg. Have extra hacksaw blades available. When both bones are divided, have your assistant drop the amputated extremity into the bucket and chuck it overboard.

13. Find the major arteries as shown in figure 26. If you do not locate them easily, let your second assistant release the tourniquet slightly. Watch for the spurting vessels and sew them shut. Use a simple running stitch. If you do not have suture materials, use sailmaker's twine and needles from your sail repair kit. Vessels must be sewn; if you simply tie strings around them, they may slip off. Sew tightly.

14. When you have secured the major vessels, again release the tourniquet a little to find other bleeding. Sew all the lesser vessels shut or sew muscle bundles together over them.

15. When bleeding is stopped except for a slight oozing, spread a generous amount of antibiotic ointment over the amputated stump. Do not close the skin.
16. Place Vaseline or plain gauze on top of the antibiotic ointment.
17. Add handfuls of gauze to cover the stump. Wrap firmly with Ace bandages (two or three).
18. Using the following method, make two adhesive traction strips and stick them to the skin on each side of the leg above the dressing: Cut a 1-foot strip of 3-inch adhesive tape and, doubling back 3 inches, stick tape to itself. Make a second strip the same way. Apply antiseptic compound to the stump and allow it to dry. Then stick adhesive strips to each side of the stump for use in traction.
19. Move the patient to his bunk. Fasten the traction strips to line through a block to a weight of about two pounds. This exerts a gentle traction. It makes the patient more comfortable and prevents retraction of soft tissues.

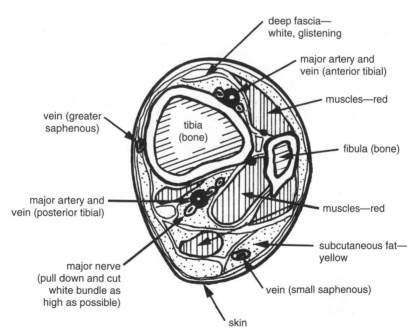

Fig. 26. Cross section through left lower leg

FOLLOW-UP CARE OF AMPUTATION

1. Control pain with Demerol 75–100 mg by injection every three or four hours as necessary for the first few days. Pain will diminish until Tylenol #3 by mouth will suffice.
2. Change dressings as infrequently as possible—only when they become soiled or wet. However, the wound should be checked carefully for infection every two days. It is easier and more comfortable for the patient if the dressings are first soaked with sterile (boiled) water that has been cooled to room temperature. This will loosen the debris and healing area from the bandages.
3. See instructions for general patient care in chapters 2 and 3.
4. Give Keflex 500 mg four times daily or Cipro 500 mg two times daily for ten days or until clean healing develops. This will be indicated by less discharge and pink healthy tissues when wound is dressed.
5. Tetanus 0.5 mg booster should be given.
6. Leave a tourniquet loosely around the lower thigh at all times. If bleeding occurs, cinch it up until you can get organized to control it by pressure or by local anesthesia injection and resuturing of the bleeding vessel.

Discussion of Amputation

The gangrenous extremity furnishes excellent soil for deadly bacterial growth while its connections to the living parts above provide excellent channels to spread infection; unchecked it can prove fatal. The amputation removes this culture medium. The wide-open stump allows adequate drainage of any infection that has already reached the lymph vessels and tissue spaces in the living parts above.

It is easier to amputate the leg below, rather than through, the knee. First, it is difficult to cut through the knee joint accurately, and second, the cartilage on the proximal joint surface must be chiseled away—a tedious process. Below-the-knee amputations with salvage of the joint cause considerably less disability than those which sacrifice the joint.

Skin traction applied immediately after operation and held until healing is complete assures adequate soft tissue (muscle and fascia) to provide a good stump—one that can be fitted with an artificial limb.

This procedure can be adapted to amputations of the forearm below the elbow. Follow the same steps, and the anatomy is reasonably similar.

Delayed amputation (application of permanent tourniquet and ice pack to limb beyond) is really a physiological removal of the limb, i.e., it is externalized completely from the body. This controls infection unless it ascends beyond the tourniquet and invades the leg above, but this is rarely the case.

Compound Fractures, Wounds, and Amputations

Amputation will have to be done eventually by a surgeon when the patient arrives in port, once a permanent tourniquet is set. Often cold will provide enough anesthesia for the amputation with no other local or general anesthetic drug necessary.

CHAPTER 4

Burns, Administration of All Injectable Fluids

Your trawler, *Nomad,* is rolling along in a heavy following sea, halfway between Turtle Bay and Cabo San Lucas, at a comfortable 10 knots. It is 1200 hours Tuesday; the galley slave lights off the fires for lunch.

A maverick wave tosses *Nomad* onto her beam ends. There is a scream below and the cook skyrockets up the companionway, hair and clothes ablaze.

First, put out the fire. Don't get burned yourself. Roll him on the deck, wrap him in foul weather gear—anything that's handy.

He sits on the cabin floor; he shivers with fright and pain, an awesome sight—hair and eyebrows singed away, bits of burned clothing hanging on his chest and tummy. He smells like an overdone steak.

1. Be sure his airway is free and quickly assess for other injuries.
2. Control pain and fright.
    a. Cover all burned areas with cool towels, wrung out in fresh water (iced, if you have it), for three to five minutes.
    b. Give him 100 mg of Demerol by intramuscular injection (see figure 12).
3. Boil three quarts of fresh water in a covered pan for twenty minutes. Allow it to cool.
4. Scrub your hands for ten minutes with Betadine and fresh water; clean your fingernails and put on sterile gloves.
5. Remove the cold compresses and wash the burns. Use the water you have sterilized, gauze sponges, and Betadine. Clean all areas gently, but thoroughly. By now, the Demerol and cold compresses have dulled the pain.
6. When the burns are cleaned, you must now decide whether it is a serious (i.e., potentially fatal) or nonserious (painful and annoying) burn.

You determine the severity of any burn by the extent (percent) of body surface involved and the depth of injury, the latter expressed in degrees. The area (percent) of the body burned is calculated for adults from the *Rule of Nines* (see figure 27). For a child, see chapter 21, figure 54.) The illustration is self-explanatory. The depth of burn is determined by the appearance of the skin surface.

First degree—redness of skin only (see figure 29, top).

Second degree—blisters (see figure 29, center).

Third degree—skin surface dead white or brown and insensitive to pinprick (see figure 29, bottom).

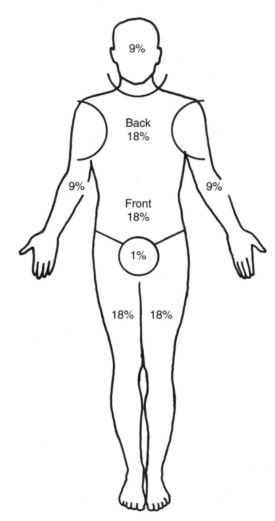

Fig. 27. *Rule of Nines:* percent of adult body area burned. (See figure 54 for children.)

You observe that your patient's scalp (5 percent of body surface) is blistered—second-degree burn. The front and back of his chest and front of his abdomen (26 percent of surface) are involved in second- and third-degree burns.

This is a serious burn (potentially lethal); the rule is if 20 percent or more of the body surface is burned to second or third degree, the burn is serious.

You may have some difficulty in applying the two determinants. Make a rough estimate of body surface involved from the chart. You may be a bit puzzled about the exact depth in a given area. Do your best. These formulae are designed as a rough guide; as such they are useful. They are about as accurate as an observation of your boat's speed by the chip log and stopwatch. To continue treatment:

7. Apply Silvadene 1% cream liberally. Cover this with sterile gauze patches and then wrap firmly with Ace bandages or KLING conforming gauze bandage. You may decide to treat the scalp by exposure if you have difficulty fastening a head bandage.
8. Call for help if you have a ship-to-shore phone. Aid may be forthcoming in a few hours or may be delayed for some days.

BURN SHOCK

The most serious early complication of a bad burn is burn shock; it may not develop for some hours or not at all, but you must be ready. Oliguria (diminished urine output) heralds the approach of serious burn shock as clearly as dark clouds on the horizon anticipate a rain squall.

9. Continue pain control with Demerol. One of the signs of over-dosage is increasing drowsiness and listlessness. In this case, you will discontinue pain injection temporarily.
10. Make several quarts of "salty lemonade" to replace the fluids and minerals lost: To 1 quart of water, add 1 level teaspoonful of table salt, a teaspoon of baking soda, and any flavoring available (lemon is best).
11. Urge your patient to drink as much of this as he can without becoming nauseated. Let him drink any fluid that he will (except alcoholic beverages), in any quantity, but urge the salty mixture.
12. As soon as practicable after injury, make the patient empty his bladder. Note the time in the ship's log; throw away the urine.
13. One hour later, have him void again; measure the amount and record this in the log at the new time. Discard the urine.
14. Do this every hour for twenty-four hours.

Let's have a look at the log:

1500—First urine discarded. Unmeasured.

1600—Urine measures 240 cc (8 ounces, one standard measuring cup).

1700—Urine = 120 cc (4 ounces, or ½ standard measuring cup).

1800—Urine = 70 cc (1¼ ounces, or slightly over ¼ cup).

Your patient has voided less than two ounces in the last hour—definite oliguria. Burn shock is on the way.

15. Post a constant watch at his bunk; offer him fluids every ten minutes. Urge him to drink anything he will take. Beer is permissible; no hard liquor.

1900—Urine = 15 cc (½ ounce, barely covers the bottom of the measuring cup).

His personal barometer indicates storms ahead: weakness, rapid pulse, sweating appear, and worst of all he begins to vomit. Now you will have to give his fluids parenterally. If you don't, his chance for survival is poor.

FLUID PREPARATION AND ADMINISTRATION

In cases of shock it is necessary to give large volumes of fluids in a short period of time. The best method for this is to use intravenous infusion. Hopefully someone aboard will be familiar with this technique. Otherwise the instructions below, adapted from the excellent material published by the U.S. Department of Health, Education, and Welfare in *The Ship's Medicine Chest and Medical Aid at Sea*, should be helpful:

Intravenous administration refers to the introduction of sterile solutions directly into a vein (see figure 27A). Giving a large quantity of solution is referred to as an infusion.

Injection of sterile medication into a vein is indicated when rapid absorption is desired. An infusion of a sterile solution is started when fluids cannot be taken by mouth.

Veins of the inner aspect of the elbow generally are used for the administration of intravenous solutions. These veins are easy to reach, tend to be quite superficial, are fairly large, and are well supported by muscular and connective tissue. Veins on the back of the hand and at the ankle sometimes are used, but they are more difficult to enter and tend to roll easily.

Either arm may be used for intravenous therapy. If the patient is right-handed and both arms appear to be equally usable, the left arm is selected usually so that the right arm is free for the patient's use.

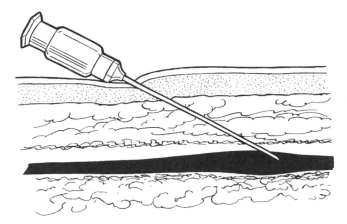

Fig. 27A. Intravenous injection.

Always make sure that sterile technique is used when a vein is being entered. When performing an intravenous infusion, this procedure should be followed:

- Assemble equipment–container of parenteral fluid or IV solution, administration set, needle (20 or 21-gauge, 1½ inch or 2 inches), prepackaged alcohol sponges, tourniquet, stand for IV container, arm board.
- Remove the protective covering and the rubber diaphragm from the solution's bottle.
- Remove the administration set from the package. Remove the protective cover from the spike, and insert the spike into the administration site of the bottle.
- Remove the protective cover from the end of the administration set. Invert the bottle so that the solution flows into the drip chamber and through the tubing.
- When the tubing is completely full of solution, close the slide clamp.
- Place the needle onto the end of the tubing, being careful to maintain aseptic technique. (Some administration sets come with the needle already attached.)
- Hang the IV from any fixture on the cabin overhead, several feet above the infusion site.
- Cut several pieces of one-half inch tape.
- Place the patient's arm on a board with a tourniquet under the arm, about 1½ inches above the intended site of entry. Secure the arm to the board with a bandage.

- Apply the tourniquet about two inches above the site of the infusion and direct the ends away from the site of the injection.
- Ask the patient to open and close his or her fist. Observe and palpate for a suitable vein.
- Cleanse the skin thoroughly with an alcohol sponge at and around the site of the injection.
- Use the thumb to retract down the vein and the soft tissue about two inches below the intended site of injection.
- Hold the needle at a 45° angle with the bevel up in line with the vein (see figure 27B) and directly alongside the wall of the vein at a point about one-half inch away from the intended site of venipuncture. Allow the fluid to enter the needle and drip out. *(This will remove all the air from the tubing, in order to prevent an air embolism.)* Then clamp the tube and proceed.
- Insert the needle through the skin, lower the angle of the needle until nearly parallel with the skin, following the same course as the vein, and insert it into the vein.
- When blood comes back through the needle, open the pinch clamp and insert the needle three-fourths of an inch to one inch farther into the vein.
- Release the tourniquet.
- Open the clamp on the infusion tube.
- Tape the needle securely in place (see figure 27C).
- *Regulate the rate of flow (drops per minute) carefully.* Observe at frequent intervals to prevent variance in flow and to see that it is stopped before all the solution is administered *(to prevent air from entering the vein).* The number of drops per ml will vary with different administration sets. This information will be found

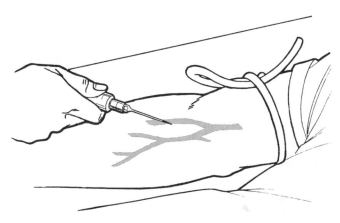

Fig. 27B. Site of an intravenous injection.

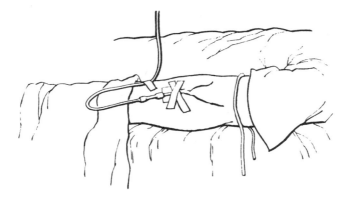

Fig. 27C. Intravenous injection procedure.

on the administration set packaging. For example, if the set delivered 15 drops per ml, and it is desired that 1000 ml of solution be administered in a five-hour period, the rate of flow would be about 50 drops per minute.

• Anchor the arm on an arm board.
• One of the drawbacks of this technique is that the needle may infiltrate normal tissue, that is, get out of the vein. The fluid will not be absorbed well with the needle in this abnormal position, causing pain to the patient. In a rolling ship keeping the IV in place can be challenging. Observe frequently the site of the infusion to detect puffiness of tissue (indicating swelling from infiltration of the solution into the tissues. *If present, discontinue the intravenous infusion and restart in another vein, using another sterile needle.*

An alternative technique, first described in 1913, is that of hypodermoclysis, that is, giving fluids subcutaneously (under the skin, directly into fatty tissues). The primary sites to use are the front of either thigh or the upper chest wall. In the past fifty years, this technique has rarely been used except in pediatric cases where obtaining a good vein for intravenous therapy was extremely difficult. However, in 1996, an extensive review of the world's medical literature over the preceding thirty years, disclosed the following:

a. Hypodermoclysis is easy to set up and maintain, improving patient comfort and mobility. For shipborne travel, this is a real plus.
b. With no medically experienced person aboard, this method offers an effective and relatively risk-free way to administer fluids.

c. Over a twelve-hour period 1000 cc should be given. This allows for better absorption and less pain to the patient.

The same solution, that is 5% Dextrose Ringer's Lactate, is appropriate for IV or the "clysis" technique. This is preferable to trying to make your own solution at sea. If you are using the subcutaneous method, here is how you proceed:

Hang the filled DRL outfit bottle above the patient's bunk; insert the needle into the patient's thigh. Open the clamp on the tubing and let the fluid run in under the skin (see figure 28). The leg will swell; it may be moderately painful.

Insert a Foley catheter into the patient's bladder (see chapter 6 for technique) and leave in-lying. This enables you to measure hourly urine output more accurately in a very ill patient. Open the catheter clamp each hour to measure urine output. For urine output and fluids to be given to a child, see chapter 21, "Treatment of a Severely Burned Child (Special Problems) . . ."

Continue the log of the burned galley worker:

2000—Urine = a few drops only from the catheter. Patient pale, clammy, sweating, and dull; pulse rapid.

16. The subcutaneous fluid swells at the right thigh at the site of the original injection (one quart of solution has been given). Move the needle to the left thigh and attach a second DRL.

2100—Urine = ½ ounce; patient is confused and irrational.
2200—Urine = same; patient's condition is unchanged.
2300—Urine = ½ ounce.
2400—Urine = 1 ounce; patient is still drowsy and weak.
0100—Urine = ¾ ounce; patient is restless.
0200—Urine = 1½ ounces; patient is restless and semiconscious, but responds to questions.
0300—Urine = 2½ ounces; patient is less sweaty, more responsive.
0400—Urine = 3 ounces; patient is definitely more alert; has had 3 quarts of solution.
0500—Urine = 3 ounces; nausea subsides; drinks some fluid.
0600—Urine = 4 ounces; drinking well; weakness gone and completely alert.
0700—Urine = 8 ounces; patient thirsty and mildly hungry. Give him food and drink. Stop subcutaneous fluids.

Make no mistake—you have saved his life. Without your parenteral fluids he would not have made it through the night.

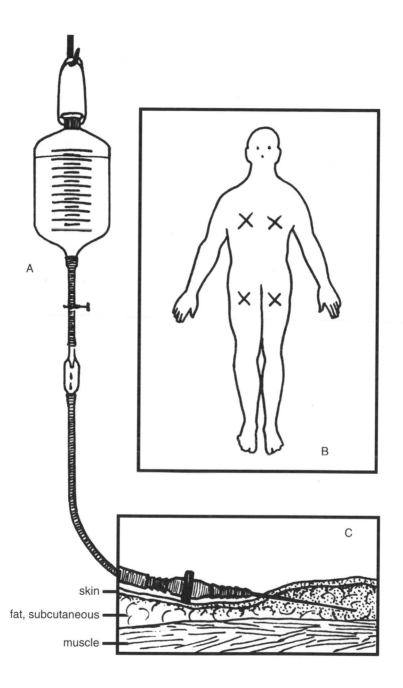

Fig. 28. (A) 5% DRL, 1,000 cc (includes plastic tubing and needle), (B) Sites for fluid injection, (C) Position of subcutaneous needle.

17. Remove the catheter.
18. The situation is under control. From now on you will have to change dressings every other day. Give Demerol 100 mg forty-five minutes beforehand; remove the dirty dressings and replace with clean. Should you run out of dressings, leave the last one in place until it becomes too objectionable by sight and smell; then remove it and simply expose the burned area to the air.
19. Give Keflex 500 mg, four times a day to combat the skin infection and that of deeper tissues that so often occurs. A tetanus booster of 0.5 ml is also required.
20. Feed your patient. You have treated a major burn and one that developed the most dreaded early complication—shock. You will turn him over to a physician's care in good condition and have reason to be proud.

Discussion of Burns

Burns may vary from minor annoyances to fatal injuries. Often the severity is immediately obvious but many times it is not. For example, a third-degree burn of the entire trunk (36 percent of body surface) is a serious injury.

The patient may not appear ill at first. There is little pain—the deep burn destroys the nerves to the skin. Pain will develop later when the surrounding parts swell up.

It is important, then, to use the Rule of Nines (adults) and the depth of burn to determine soon after injury what you must expect to treat. It is useful also in terms of your cruise plans.

Often a burn that looks frightening (blisters of the entire front of the chest) is not serious. It is 9 percent of body surface, second degree. Treat locally with Neosporin antibiotic ointment, a bandage, and something for pain, and in a couple of weeks it will be healed.

First-degree burns (redness only) are rarely important. Sunburn causes most of them. This is painful and annoying but local treatment with cooling compresses together with Tylenol #3, will control the pain. First-degree burns of over 80 percent of the body surface can become serious and should be carefully watched for development of oliguria. If this occurs, treat the patient as though you were dealing with a deeper burn.

Certain other burns are serious because of the structures involved, even though less than 20 percent of the body surface may be burned. Burns about the mouth, throat, and face may swell and interfere with breathing and swallowing. If an open airway is threatened by such swelling, pass the resuscitating tube through the mouth and throat before they close. If swallowing becomes too difficult, administer fluids parenterally.

Third-degree burns of an extremity (foot, hand, etc.), although small in size, can cause serious trouble—burned tissues may form the starting place for an overwhelming infection in a few days. Antibiotics help prevent this. And such a local burn will be less likely to become infected if dried out by air exposure. This is why a burned extremity is best treated by exposure.

Burns about the rectum or the genitals are also dangerous—the former because it is almost impossible to prevent a burn near the rectum from becoming infected from bowel movements. Give the patient with a perirectal burn three tablets of Lomotil three times daily to prevent bowel movements. It is possible for the human animal to go for weeks without a bowel movement and this avoids infecting the burn. If a fecal impaction forms, this can be treated later.

A burn near the genitals can cause the patient to retain urine—in a male, the penis may swell so that voiding urine is not possible. If a urogenital burn causes retention, catheterization is necessary.

TREATMENT OF BURNS

The modern treatment of burn wounds is described in detail in chapter 21. It is similar for adult or child.

Burn shock, which is the deadliest part of any burn in the first few days, is primarily due to loss of water and salts from the bloodstream. Protein is also lost but there is little one can do about that on shipboard, so we will concentrate on the former.

Oozing from the burns and swelling of the nearby tissues suck fluid from the bloodstream in surprising amounts—four to five quarts each twenty-four hours in a moderate-size burn.

The lost fluid slows the blood circulation through the kidneys; this produces oliguria (reduced urine output) which anticipates shock. Hospitals everywhere measure urine output to anticipate the onset of burn shock and to judge the success of fluid therapy. A modern hospital will study many other parameters of body function when treating a severe burn, but measurement of urine output is the most useful at sea.

The other symptoms of burn shock—apprehension, weakness, pallor, nausea, and vomiting—will appear later, but do not wait for these to develop. Replace the fluid; judge your success at this by the urine output—try to keep it above 2 ounces per hour (see chapter 21 for a child's urine output)—and your patient will survive the initial injury.

The subcutaneous method of giving the parenteral fluid is one of many. It assumes that you will have 5% DRL with tubing, drip bulb, and sterile needle in your first aid kit. These materials can be obtained from any surgical supply house.

You may choose, if you have adequate storage space, to buy prepared quart bottles of salt solution. These are sterile and come complete with tubing, needles, and printed instructions for their use. For a long cruise (three to six months) half a dozen might be useful. Other conditions (diarrhea, dehydration, heat exhaustion) need them.

If you wish to administer fluids by a more rapid method (intravenously, instead of subcutaneously), discuss this with your family physician before you start out. The fluids and equipment are similar; the difference lies in technique. The subcutaneous method described on p. 67 is learned easily by anyone in five minutes and is almost foolproof. The insertion of a needle into a vein for intravenous administration is more difficult and hazardous. Perhaps you will have someone aboard familiar with it.

Crush injury, bleeding, and major infection, such as peritonitis, may also cause shock. The symptoms of pallor, rapid pulse, low blood pressure (less than 90 mm), sweating, and apprehension or dullness, plus oliguria, will diagnose the condition. Treat this as you did the burn shock. In addition, if there is high fever (104°F or above), give Decadron (adrenal cortical extract) ampules, one by injection every twelve hours for four doses.

Dry skin, pounding slow pulse, high or normal blood pressure, plus oliguria, denote merely simple dehydration and not shock.

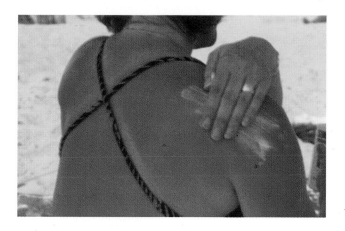

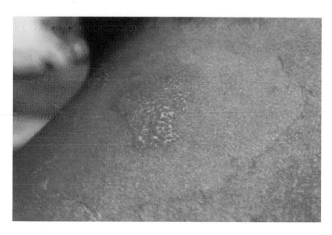

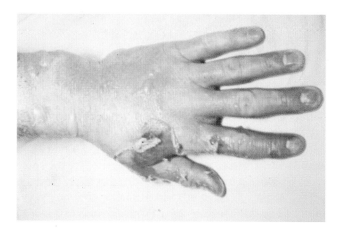

Fig. 29. *Top,* First-degree burn: redness of skin and swelling. *Center,* Second-degree burn: blisters and redness. *Bottom,* Third-degree burn: loss of skin, anesthetic to pinprick. Photos © Contributor/Custom Medical Stock Photo.

CHAPTER 5

Heat Exhaustion, Heatstroke, and Seasickness

HEAT EXHAUSTION

An April cruise from New York to Barbados puts your cruising ketch, *Restless,* six days out of port heading to warmer waters. All has gone well; you have been reaching all the way and the cold you are leaving behind makes your crew content to stand all watches, even the midwatch, with no complaints.

On the sixth day out, the air temperature rises to 85°F at 1200 hours and the relative humidity is 85 percent. Trouble descends upon you like a flight of locusts. Next morning, your port watch captain complains his group has had more than their fair share of night watches and dirty duties.

You review the log with him, point out that this is not entirely true and that it will all even up before you arrive at your destination. The starboard watch captain stands beside you and takes a haughty attitude toward his shipmate's complaints. This does not ease the tension.

You finally straighten it out and the crew goes back to work grumbling. Serenity and joy have left your cruise. Discussion spreads until everyone is griping at everyone else in a way that makes you wish you had never planned a spring cruise.

Thunderheads build up along the horizon. On the eighth day at 1600 hours, a sudden squall demands a sail change. The port watch captain goes forward to lower the Genoa. He hauls the huge sail onto the foredeck as the halyard is paid out; suddenly he collapses.

Others salvage him and the sail. They carry him to his bunk. He lies there gray of face, so weak he can barely fill his lungs with air.

Examine him:

1. His skin is wet and clammy,
2. His eyes are sunken into their sockets,
3. His pulse at the wrist is hardly perceptible. If you take his blood pressure, you find it low.
4. His oral temperature is 97.8°F, one degree below normal.

You diagnose heat exhaustion. You know now that your whole crew, challenged by heat and humid weather, has suffered a milder form of this disorder. It explains the generally rotten dispositions you encountered in the past few days.

But your port watch captain is sick. The others are merely uncomfortable.

1. Wipe him dry with towels.
2. Make two quarts of salty lemonade as described for burns (see chapter 4) and have him sip this.
3. Give him two enteric-coated salt tablets plus a glass of water with each.
4. Keep him warm, covering him with sheets and blankets if necessary.
5. Keep him at rest in his bunk.
6. If he retains the fluids given by mouth, he should be feeling better in an hour or two. Continue the salty lemonade, but now he may have a cup of hot coffee or tea.
7. Give him two enteric-coated salt tablets every four hours until he has had six tablets.
8. If he vomits, stop oral fluids; give him a Phenergan rectal suppository. Wait half an hour, then start oral salty fluids again.
9. If he vomits again, administer parenterally salt solution as described for use in the treatment of burn shock (see chapter 4). Give him two or three quarts of this intravenously or subcutaneously as rapidly as he will absorb it. If using subcutaneous route, change injection sites frequently.
10. Avoid non-salt-containing fluids except for the cup or two of coffee or tea.
11. If the patient does not recover, cardiac stimulants will probably be of little value, but must be considered along with parenteral Decadron (cortisone therapy). This gets pretty tricky and it is advisable to consult with a physician by radiotelephone.
12. You will judge the success of your treatment by his response. He will feel stronger, his pulse will firm up and become slower, and he will sweat, but his body will feel warmer to the touch.
13. When he recovers, have him resume his regular duties gradually.

To protect the others, have the galley crew salt all chow heavily and keep enteric-coated salt tablets handy. Anyone who feels weak and excessively sweaty should take a tablet or two with plenty of water. These measures will prevent severe heat exhaustion and improve dispositions as well.

Another sign of impending heat exhaustion is heat cramps. These occur in the abdominal or leg muscles and come on quite suddenly. They may last a short while or be quite persistent, and indicate a need for more salt intake.

HEATSTROKE

Your Barbados cruise has further unpleasant surprises in store. At 1200 hours the twelfth day out you are trying to rest below decks away from the 100°F heat and the hot sunlight. There is a sudden yell for you from topside.

You dash up the ladder just in time to see the helmsman slump forward and let the wheel spin. A watch mate grabs it and brings the boat back on course.

"What's the matter?" you ask the fallen shipmate.

"I'm hot and dizzy and my head is pounding like the devil," he says. He slithers onto the cockpit floor and passes out.

Examination shows:

1. He is unconscious.
2. His skin is dry.
3. He is not sweating.
4. His forehead is hot to your touch and livid red in color.
5. His pulse is full and bounding.

You recognize heatstroke. Treatment is urgent.

1. Get him below, out of the sun, at once.
2. Log his rectal temperature; if it is below 103°F, cool him gradually with alcohol or cool water sponges. If his temperature is over 103°F (and likely it will be), heroic measures are necessary. Strip him naked and sluice him down with buckets of cold or ice water.
3. Log successive rectal temperatures every thirty minutes; when it drops below 102°F, stop the cooling measures.
4. Dry him off and put him in his bunk with a light covering.
5. If he becomes irrational, delirious, or hyperactive, give Valium 10 mg by injection.
6. As he begins to recover, give him food and nonalcoholic fluid as he wishes.
7. Give Tylenol #3 or two tablets of aspirin every three to four hours as necessary for headache.
8. When his headache subsides and his temperature has been normal for twenty-four hours, allow him to resume his normal activities.

9. Put him on night watches for the rest of the cruise and keep him below deck, as cool as possible, and out of the sun in the daytime.

Discussion

Heat exhaustion and heatstroke represent failures in the physiological mechanisms that dissipate heat. Each condition deranges different body defenses and produces a different, though related, group of symptoms.

The body needs water for all its functions including heat loss. Daily requirements under ordinary conditions are:

1. 1000 cc to moisten air breathed,
2. 500 cc for minimal or insensible perspiration (perspiration that is so slight as to pass unnoticed, but is always present),
3. 1000 cc for urine excretion.

This water is obtained from:

1. Liquids and semisolid foods (lean cooked meat, for example, is 60–70 percent water),
2. Oxygenation (burning) of carbohydrate, protein, and fat in body metabolism: 100 gm fat burned furnishes 107 gm water; 100 gm carbohydrate burned furnishes 55 gm water; 100 gm protein burned furnishes 41 gm water.

The body also requires certain minerals; the chief one for purposes of this discussion is sodium chloride or ordinary table salt. The average 150-pound man on the usual diet will excrete at least 2.5 gm of sodium chloride in urine and sweat daily. This amount has to be replaced since the body cannot manufacture it.

Much greater amounts of salt and water may be lost with exercise during warm humid weather. A football player, for instance, may lose 1400–1500 cc of water and 3–5 gm of salt in one hour's play on a warm September day.

Water replacement alone will not suffice. Salt must also be taken in. The body is a chemical machine and homeostatic mechanisms of infinite complexity operate continuously to maintain the concentration of electrolytes (in this case, salt) constant, since within reasonable limits it is the concentration of electrolytes rather than the absolute amount present that determines chemical activity. If total body salt content is low, the kidneys will excrete body water to restore normal concentration. If water is given by mouth without salt when the salt stores of the body are depleted, the water will be excreted at once.

The salt and water carry heat via the bloodstream from the internal cells of the body where it is manufactured to the lungs and skin surface where it can be lost. It is similar to the transport of heat in your automobile engine from the block to the radiator.

When salt and water are lost through excessive perspiration due to work in a hot and humid atmosphere, the total volume of body fluids is diminished. If plain water is drunk, it is not retained. Eventually such fluid losses reduce the volume of blood circulating until a shocklike state develops, somewhat similar to that following a severe burn. This shock state lowers body metabolism and body temperature since oxygen transport to the tissues is diminished. Hence the person suffering from heat exhaustion feels week, his body is cold and clammy, his temperature subnormal, his blood pressure low, and his urine output is low. Treatment provides salt and fluid to restore the circulating volume.

Heatstroke, a much more dangerous condition, results when the external environment prevents heat loss from the lungs and skin. Extremely high air temperature, or moderately high temperature plus excessive humidity, creates this climate. The temperature of the blood rises. This in turn knocks out the sensitive heat control center at the base of the brain. The blood vessels to the skin close down (vasoconstrict), sweating stops, and so does heat loss.

The person with heatstroke, as you noted, was hot and did not sweat. Headache, elevated blood pressure, delirium, convulsions, coma, and death proceed in rapid order with true heatstroke.

The treatment is external body cooling. If the temperature is moderately elevated, this may be gradual. If the temperature is above 103° F, it must be rapid and heroic. Valium, 5–10 mg by injection, helps control convulsions or delirium.

The thoughtful skipper protects the crew from heatstroke and heat exhaustion by anticipation. The cruise will be more enjoyable too, because such measures prevent development of a minor degree of heat exhaustion that causes general grouchiness.

External temperatures of 80°F, with a relative humidity of 50 percent or over, sound the alert. A wet and dry bulb thermometer records humidity. It is a must for hot weather or tropical cruising. The relative humidity is important because the more saturated the air with water vapor, the less evaporation and cooling occur on the body surface. To further our analogy, it would be like submerging the car radiator in a steam bath and expecting it to lose heat rapidly.

The first few days of exposure to this type of atmosphere are the most dangerous. After a short period of time, the body acclimatizes to increases of heat and humidity by:

1. Dilation of the blood vessels in the skin with greater surface radiant heat loss.
2. Increased perspiration with low salt content: more evaporative cooling, and body salt stores are saved.
3. Increasing total body fluid volume to implement these mechanisms.
4. Decreasing excretion of salt in the urine.

Athletic trainers and coaches know acclimatization takes from five to fifteen days. Therefore, during the first warm weeks of football season, workouts are kept at a minimum, extra water and salt are made available, and light clothing is worn. In addition, practice sessions are planned to some degree according to daily variations of temperature and humidity.

In 1988 a fleet of native craft sailed from Bali to Darwin, Australia. On the first leg of the journey, a young Japanese sailor staggered from his boat with obvious heat exhaustion. In addition to the usual recommendations, a doctor following the event told him to immerse his hat hourly for the rest of the trip to cool his head. On arriving in Darwin, the young sailor said that he had followed the instructions and felt that without that simple advice he would not have completed the two-thousand-mile trip.

When you first reach a subtropical climate with a crew that is unacclimatized, you should:

1. Have everyone wear light protective clothing, headgear, and sunglasses that protect from the sun.
2. Shorten daytime watch hours—two on and two off, instead of four on and four off—during the heat of the day.
3. Have frequent cooling sessions on deck. Sluice members of the watch with a bucket of seawater from time to time, or rig a shower with a grill placed in the bottom of a sea anchor. This frequent cooling is similar to spot coolers on merchant and naval ships. In the engine rooms, huge blowers blast cool air and, from time to time, members of the engine room gang stand under one. It enables them to tolerate otherwise unbearable temperature and humidity.
4. Provide adequate fluids in the diet, and plenty of carbohydrates; protein should be avoided, since its ingestion is followed by increased body heat.
5. Provide enteric-coated salt tablets. They dissolve only in the small intestine, are absorbed more rapidly, and do not cause vomiting with high salt concentration in the stomach.

SEASICKNESS

A wise skipper leaves the persistently seasick ashore when embarking on a long ocean race or cruise. It is hard to do for many reasons, not the least of which is that such folk will often hide this weakness in the hope of being asked to go along.

Drugs will control seasickness but too often substitute drowsiness. If a crewperson depends on drugs for the long haul, you may wind up coddling a sleepy sloucher while all hands double up to stand his watches. Many sailors suffer mild seasickness at the start of a voyage but acquire sea legs in a day or two. These make good crewmen; the steadily seasick do not. Unusual weather conditions (windless for several hours in a huge ground swell) may induce the hardiest sailor to lose his lunch. If vomiting continues, he will lose his vigor and interest in the cruise as well.

Seasickness is a motion sickness caused by repetitive angular and linear acceleration and deceleration, and characterized primarily by nausea and vomiting. Excessive stimulation of the inner ear by motion is the primary cause. Individuals' susceptibility varies greatly. It also appears that there is a genetic predisposition, with Oriental people being especially troubled by seasickness. Visual stimuli (for example, moving horizon), poor ventilation, fumes, smoke, and carbon monoxide, and emotional factors, for example, fear and anxiety, commonly act in concert with motion to precipitate an attack. Nausea and vomiting are characteristic of this condition. This may be preceded by yawning, hyperventilation, salivation, pallor, profuse cold sweating, and somnolence. Aerophagia (an abnormal swallowing of air), dizziness, headache, a general discomfort, and fatigue may also occur.

Once nausea and vomiting develop, the patient is weak and unable to concentrate. However, with prolonged exposure to motion, individuals may adapt and gradually return to well-being. But symptoms may be reinitiated by more severe motion or recurrence of motion after a short respite. Prolonged motion sickness with vomiting may lead to hypotension, dehydration, and depression. Motion sickness can be a serious complication in patients who are ill from other causes.

Susceptible individuals should minimize exposure by positioning themselves where there is the least motion, for example, amidships. A supine or semirecumbent position with the head braced may help matters. Reading should be avoided. A well-ventilated cabin is important, and going out on deck to sit in the fresh air is helpful. Alcoholic or dietary excesses before traveling may increase the likelihood of seasickness. Small amounts of fluids and simple food should be taken frequently during extended periods of exposure.

Phenergan 25 mg rectal suppositories will usually control the nausea and vomiting. This drug, one of the most reliable and easily used remedies for seasickness, is best given one hour before going to sea, but may be administered at any time and repeated every eight to twelve hours. If the sufferer is unable to retain salt and water after this drug, prepare and administer salt solution parenterally as described for burn shock in chapter 4. Scopalomine, which is usually delivered via a dermal patch, has shown significant side effects in many people and is not recommended.

There are many other remedies that have helped some people, including aromatherapy using peppermint oil and ginger. Ginger root capsules may provide relief. Acupressure over the wrist in the region of the radial artery may be helpful; wristbands are sold without a prescription that provide pressure in this area.

CHAPTER 6

Abdominal Pain and Genitourinary Emergencies

One day as you cruise 1,000 miles from the nearest port, you note one of your crew skips morning chow. File it in the back of your mind for attention later on in the day.

He passes up a second meal. Ask him why he is not eating.

"Got a stomachache," he says, "but it isn't bad."

1. Do not accept this evaluation. Take him someplace remote from the wisecracks of the rest of the crew and ask:
   a. Did pain or nausea start first?
   b. Where is the pain? How bad is it, really?
   c. Has it changed its location since it began?
   d. Do you feel like vomiting?
   e. Is it getting worse or better?
   f. Does walking make your stomach hurt? If so, where?
   g. Have you ever had a pain like it before?
2. Have him lie flat on his back with his whole abdomen exposed.
3. Rub your hands to warm them; gently, with palms flat, press each of the four abdominal quadrants, right and left upper and lower. Note any tender areas (see figure 30).
4. Take his temperature.
5. Log the above findings in detail.
6. Insert one Dulcolax rectal suppository if the patient says that he may be seriously constipated.

If his pain persists another twelve hours:

1. Get him off his feet.
2. Allow only water, tea, or coffee without cream or sugar by mouth.
3. Repeat your examination now and every six hours (history, oral temperature, abdominal palpation). Log all observations.
4. Continue above measures until appetite returns, temperature becomes normal, pain stops, and the abdomen is not tender at all. Then he may get up and go to duty.

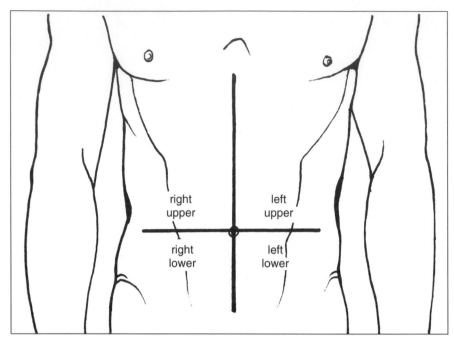

Fig. 30. Abdominal examination: the four quadrants.

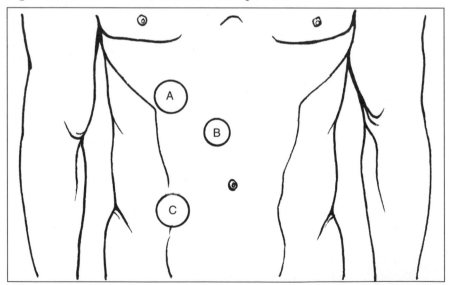

Fig. 31. Abdominal tenderness: (A) acute cholecystitis, (B) simple duodenal ulcer, (C) acute appendicitis. These are areas that are "classically" tender in the diseases mentioned. Unfortunately there can be wide variations in the significance of this tenderness, and these are only part of the clinical picture being developed.

If, on the other hand, an examination six hours later discovers:

1. Persistent nausea or vomiting,
2. Worse pain in the abdomen,
3. The pain has shifted to the right lower abdomen and stays there (see figure 31),
4. Rebound tenderness, right lower abdomen (this is a sharp stab of pain when firm hand pressure on the abdomen is suddenly released),
5. Fever, temperature 99°F or higher,
6. Walking or jumping on the right foot causes pain in the right lower abdomen.

If symptoms 1 through 6 inclusive are present, suspect acute appendicitis—probably unruptured as yet.

If 1, 2, and 5 are present but tenderness is in the upper abdomen, acute gallbladder inflammation (cholecystitis), duodenal ulcer, or some other disease is present (see figure 32).

The following treatment is effective for painful surgical abdominal disease at this stage, whatever the underlying cause:

1. Give clear liquids only by mouth (water, tea; no milk or sugar).
2. Inject Demerol, 75–100 mg (adjust dose for child) every three to four hours as needed to control pain.
3. Keep the patient in his bunk except to use the head.
4. Give Cipro 500 mg three times daily for a minimum of five days.

The patient may improve (less pain and tenderness in the abdomen, nausea subsides, temperature becomes normal) in twenty-four to thirty-six hours and he will be well in a few days with such treatment. When you are sure all pain, abdominal tenderness, and fever are gone, feed him and put him back to duty.

If, instead, he gets worse (more pain, vomiting, abdominal distension, more tenderness and rebound tenderness, temperature 101–103°F, pulse one hundred per minute or more), the infection is spreading from its original focus to invade the peritoneal cavity. This is peritonitis (see figure 32).

Maximum tenderness in right lower abdomen suggests a ruptured appendix; tenderness and muscle spasm all over the abdomen suggest a perforated ulcer; local signs in right upper abdomen point to acute cholecystitis.

You treat peritonitis from whatever source as follows:

1. Discontinue giving Cipro.

2. Give Rocephin by deep intramuscular injection, 2 gm daily.
3. Give 1500 cc salt solution by IV or subcutaneous injection (see chapter 4).
4. Measure and record during the first twenty-four hours of treatment (measuring cup = 8 ounces = 240 cc; coffee cup also 8 ounces):
   a. IV or subcutaneous fluid actually given,
   b. Liquids drunk,
   c. Urine output,
   d. Oral loss by vomiting or nasogastric tube suction (see step 7).

You should have a fluid balance log like this:

Intake

Salt solution actually absorbed by patient	1300 cc
Sips of water by mouth	1000 cc
Total fluid intake in twenty-four hours	2300 cc

Output

Urine	800 cc
Vomited	100 cc
Total fluid output in twenty-four hours	900 cc

4. To compute fluid needs for next (second) twenty-four hours:

Basic daily requirement salt solution	1500 cc
Add left over from first day (unable to give it all) =	300 cc
	1800 cc
Subtract liquids drunk	−1000 cc
	800 cc

Give in the second twenty-four hours by intravenous or subcutaneous injection: 800 cc 5% DRL.

5. Compute fluid requirement each twenty-four hours as shown above. Fifteen hundred cc daily basic salt solution is required each twenty-four hours, plus amount equal to loss by vomiting or stomach suction (see step 7), minus water drunk during preceding twenty-four hours.
6. If urine output drops below 500 cc during any twenty-four-hour period, raise basic daily salt solution from 1500 cc to 2000 cc each twenty-four hours by subcutaneous injection.
7. Should the patient vomit repeatedly, pass a nasogastric tube. This rests the bowel. To pass a nasogastric tube:
   a. Clean your hands and put on surgical gloves.

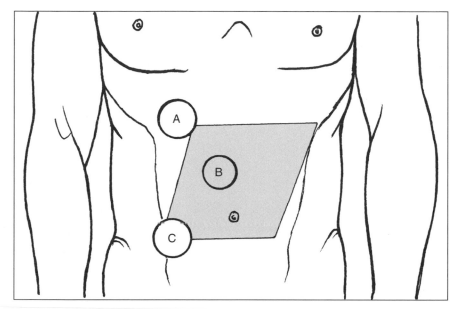

Fig. 32. Spread of tenderness and spasm, originating at: (A) ruptured gallbladder (rare), (B) perforated ulcer, (C) ruptured appendix. This is peritonitis.

b. Assemble stomach tube, lubricant, bulb syringe.
c. Sit the patient upright in his bunk.
d. Lubricate tip of nasogastric tube (Vaseline, salad oil, etc.).
e. Give the patient a cup of water to hold in his right hand.
f. Insert the tip of tube into one nostril; point it down towards
   the floor of the nose cavity.
g. Push it steadily into his nose.
h. Have patient swallow water from the cup in his hand when
   the tube hits the back of his throat.
i. Keep pushing the tube; have him keep swallowing. You will
   feel the tube hang up a bit at the cardio-esophageal junction
   (where the gullet or esophagus joins the stomach). Then it
   will pop into the stomach. The mark on the tube shows when
   it is in the stomach.
j. Tape the tube to his forehead. Check the position in the stomach by suction on the tube with the bulb syringe. You should
   get back some bile stained greenish yellow or whitish acid-
   smelling stomach fluid.

Passing the stomach tube is often not this easy. After a swallow of
water, the patient will retch, the tube will come flying out of his mouth

along with a quart or so of vomit. Never mind; you have emptied the stomach—not as neatly as you might wish—but effectively. Rest a moment; pull the tube from his nose and start over. If the patient takes a few deep breaths and makes vigorous efforts at swallowing, you will usually get the tube into the stomach. When you finally get it in place, vomiting will stop.

      k. Keep the stomach empty by suction with the bulb syringe or hang the end of the nasogastric tube into a basin on deck. Siphonage will keep emptying stomach secretion.

If the tube drains correctly, the stomach will be empty and then the patient will not vomit. If the tube plugs up, clear it by injection of one ounce of water with bulb syringe. It may improve drainage to untape tube from forehead and move it up or down a few inches.

      8. If temperature recedes, pain lessens, vomiting subsides, and abdominal tenderness goes away, the patient is getting better. Remove the stomach tube when nausea subsides. Stop the parenteral salt solution when he can drink enough to keep urine output over 500 cc in twenty-four hours.

Feed him whatever he will eat when he gets hungry. Stop antibiotic injections when oral temperature has been normal for twenty-four hours. Read chapter 7, "The Use of Antibiotics."

      9. Should he get worse rather than better (higher fever, more severe pain, persistent nausea, tenderness spreading over the abdomen), continue treatment. This will keep him alive until you reach port.

Discussion—Abdominal Pain
Common causes of abdominal pain are dietary indiscretion, constipation, and gastroenteritis (commonly called intestinal flu). More serious, though fortunately less common, causes are appendicitis, acute gallbladder infection, and duodenal ulcer disease.

Constipation may cause stomachaches so that the first step in diagnosis of abdominal pain is to give the patient a rectal suppository to help relieve any constipation. Only use the suppository if there is a reasonable chance your patient has constipation. Life afloat encourages constipation. Irregular hours, inactivity, dehydration, and limited head facilities discourage crews from daily bowel movements, particularly the shy ones. On one transpacific sailboat race, we kept a paper tacked up in the head.

Each sailor checked off a daily passage. If he skipped two days, he ate an extra ration of prunes or took a cathartic. It worked well.

Gastroenteritis, or "intestinal flu," is usually caused by a virus and shows itself by nausea and diarrhea. Fever is usually not present. Treatment is rest and Lomotil to control the fluid loss from frequent bowel movements.

APPENDICITIS

A male previously well starts an attack of acute appendicitis with a moderate pain located somewhat vaguely throughout the upper abdomen. (See chapter 20 for special problems of appendicitis in children.) Nausea follows shortly. It is axiomatic that unless pain precedes nausea, appendicitis is very rarely the trouble. In a few hours, or perhaps a day or two, the pain migrates to the right lower abdomen and settles there. It becomes increasingly severe and eventually tenderness (which differs from the pain in that you must touch the patient to determine it) develops over the site of the appendix. It is located in the right lower abdomen (see figure 31).

Appendicitis starts as a minute abscess in the appendiceal wall. Too small to hurt at first, it nevertheless flashes a message back along the nerves in the bowel wall to stop further progress of all food and fluid from above. This clamps down the pylorus muscle at the outlet of the stomach. Spasm of this muscle causes the early pain in the upper abdomen during the attack of acute appendicitis.

The abscess in the appendix enlarges and begins to hurt locally; the pain moves down to the right lower quadrant of the abdomen and the overlying abdominal wall becomes sensitive to touch. The infection at this point is still localized to the appendix. The disease is not serious yet. The potential for harm is great.

It is now, while infection is still limited to the appendix, that rest, antibiotics, and control of pain with Demerol offer the best chance of curing the disease. The infection subsides; the patient gradually recovers. This is the importance of early attention to stomachaches.

Should the abscess enlarge to burst the appendiceal wall, the infection spreads throughout the abdominal cavity. This is peritonitis (see figure 32).

Rupture of the appendix is frequently followed by sudden relief of pain. For an hour or two, the patient feels much better. Shortly, however, temperature rises, nausea and vomiting recur, pain returns, and tenderness spreads outward in all directions from the original site in the right lower abdomen. The abdominal muscles harden into spasm to protect the painful gut beneath. Be sure when treating suspected acute appendicitis that sudden relief of symptoms is permanent before you stop treatment.

Should the appendix rupture, supportive treatment (rest, parenteral fluids and parenteral antibiotics, bowel rest, and pain control) offers the body's natural defenses a chance to control peritonitis. Infected bowel loops secrete an adhesive exudate and stick together to localize or "wall off" the infection into an abscess. When you reach port, a surgeon can drain this.

The foregoing describes the classic onset and course of acute appendicitis. Unfortunately, this disease is atypical as often as it is classic. Experienced surgeons often puzzle over the diagnosis.

To reiterate, the skipper's approach to the threat of acute appendicitis is to start treatment when:

1. A previously healthy sailor gets severe abdominal pain.
2. The pain lasts twelve hours or longer.
3. A rectal suppository is ineffective in producing a good bowel movement and relief.

The treatment outlined aims to prevent acute appendicitis from progressing to a ruptured appendix, although this is not always possible. It also can sustain life if this catastrophe occurs. If diagnosis is incorrect, the treatment outlined will do no harm.

Certain individuals entering into high office and a few adventurers have undergone elective surgical removal of a normal appendix prior to setting out upon their various journeys. This is possible, reasonably safe, and a matter to be settled by each individual in discussion with a physician.

MITTELSCHMERZ

One condition peculiar to women deserves special mention—mittelschmerz. Midway between two menstrual periods, the premenopausal woman ovulates. An ovum ruptures the surface of the ovary and starts its descent toward the fallopian tube for possible fertilization. Such rupture usually passes unnoticed but, on occasion, may cause sudden right-lower or left-lower (if the left ovary is ovulating) abdominal pain. If there is a bit of blood spilled into the free abdominal cavity from the rupture, this may cause lower abdominal tenderness that simulates appendicitis. It differs, though, and of prime importance is timing. It occurs ten to fifteen days after the conclusion of the last menstrual period—hence its name, middle pain, or mittelschmerz. It is sudden in onset, as might be expected, and disappears spontaneously in a day or two.

ACUTE CHOLECYSTITIS
(GALLBLADDER INFECTION)

This disease differs from acute appendicitis as follows:

1. It may be less common in men, and it is seldom seen in both sexes below the age of thirty-five years. A surgical axiom states that acute cholecystitis occurs typically in fair, fat, forty-year-old flatulent females—but don't count on that!
2. It is a recurrent disease. Sufferers have usually had prior attacks and know what to do about them.
3. It is more dramatic than acute appendicitis. The pain can send the bravest rolling to the deck in agony. The victim's skin and eyeballs may turn bright yellow. He or she may void orange-colored urine.
4. It is a less dangerous disease than acute appendicitis in spite of the melodrama of symptoms. The infected gallbladder rarely ruptures to cause peritonitis.
5. The pain and soreness start in the upper abdomen and remain there. There is no definite sequence of pain followed by nausea, as in acute appendicitis. Vomiting, however, is common.

Treatment is designed to maintain fluids, provide antibiotics, and relieve pain. Treat suspected acute cholecystitis exactly as you do suspected acute appendicitis with the addition of atropine 1/150 gr by injection every six hours for the first forty-eight hours.

Discussion—Acute Cholecystitis (Gallbladder Infection)
The gallbladder recycles water and certain important chemicals. It also helps digest fatty foods. It is a useful but not essential organ.

Bile formed in the liver consists mainly of bilirubin (a pigment derived from breakdown of red blood hemoglobin), bile salts, calcium, and cholesterol. The gallbladder receives this mixture and withdraws water plus bile salts into the blood for reuse.

When fats are eaten, the gallbladder contracts and splashes a generous dollop of concentrated bile onto them as they emerge from the stomach into the duodenum. This bile emulsifies fat for digestion. Should the gallbladder be removed surgically, the bile duct system takes over the concentrating function.

Bile in the gallbladder, for reasons presently obscure, sometimes precipitates stones of calcium, bilirubin, and cholesterol, substances normally held in solution. Such stones may move to block the narrow cystic or common ducts. In either instance, the blocked bile builds back pressure that overdistends the gallbladder.

The gallbladder contracts violently to overcome the obstruction caused by the stone plugging the duct. It is violent contraction against obstruction that causes gallbladder colic which hurts as much as any pain humans suffer. If the obstruction is in the common duct, bile backs up through the liver into the bloodstream. The patient turns yellow (jaundice), and voids orange-colored urine (bilirubinuria).

Unless the obstructing stone falls back into the gallbladder or is pushed forward through the common duct, the disease persists until a surgeon removes the stone. He usually removes the diseased gallbladder as well, to prevent formation of future stones. Laparoscopic removal of the gallbladder can very frequently be done. This highly popular technique markedly reduces hospital stay and greatly decreases postoperative pain and disability.

The sturdy gallbladder wall sustains back pressure for long periods and perforation with peritonitis due to bile is rare. Usually the stone obstructs only the cystic duct and falls back into the gallbladder with complete relief after a few days. Atropine relaxes the muscle in the gallbladder wall.

Acute cholecystitis tends to recover spontaneously rather than rupture and produce the serious complications that follow a ruptured appendix. Recovery from an attack of gallstone disease is, however, usually only temporary because stones are present and may obstruct again at any time. It is desirable for anyone with proven gallbladder disease to discuss having it surgically corrected before cruising long distances.

DUODENAL ULCER

The pain due to duodenal ulcer is located in the right upper quadrant of the abdomen and develops when the stomach is empty. A small amount of food or antacid will bring temporary relief of pain but it will recur after a varying interval.

Diagnosis of duodenal ulcer:

1. Right upper abdominal pain when stomach is empty.
2. Antacids and/or food giving temporary relief of the pain.
3. A tender spot to the right of and a bit above the belly button (see figure 31).
4. A past history of ulcer disease or of abdominal pain when the stomach was empty, but no ulcer was found upon X-ray examination. Chances are good that an ulcer was present. X-ray examination does not discover all duodenal ulcers.

Treatment of duodenal ulcer:

1. General diet—any food that does not cause indigestion.
2. Dual antibiotics are most successful. Doxycycline 100 mg two times a day with Metronidozale 250 mg three times a day may be used, or Cipro 500 mg three times a day *alone* as a second choice.
3. No smoking or alcoholic beverages.
4. Pepto-Bismol, two tablets four times a day, along with Tagamet, one tablet at bedtime.

Discussion—Duodenal Ulcer

A healthy stomach secretes just enough hydrochloric acid to digest food actually present or anticipated by sight and smell of a meal. The stomach grinds the food, mixes it with acid and enzymes, then passes this acid chyme through the pylorus into the duodenum.

The duodenal content (pancreatic and intestinal juices plus bile) is alkaline and promptly neutralizes the incoming acid chyme. This protects the duodenal mucosa which is resistant to alkali but not to acid.

The stomach of a duodenal ulcer sufferer secretes acid continually whether or not food is present in the stomach. This excess acid, unmixed with food, squirts through the pylorus, strikes the duodenal wall, and erodes the lining to form a duodenal ulcer. It is usually about one-half inch to three-quarters of an inch in diameter. It is now known that certain bacteria disrupt the normal duodenal mucosal defense and repair, making the mucosa more susceptible to the attack of the acid. The cause of acid hypersecretion may or may not be related to stress, nervous influences, and personality type.

The ulcer, once formed, hurts when bathed in acid. Food or antacids absorb the acid and give temporary relief. A bleeding ulcer filled with blood hurts very little for the same reason.

Treatment keeps food and/or antacid constantly in the stomach to soak up the acid and the antibiotics heal the ulcer.

If untreated, the ulcer may erode an artery and bleed, or even perforate the muscle coats of the duodenal wall.

For the rest of the cruise the use of antibiotics, conventional antacids, and a diet as tolerated will help the sufferer until he or she returns to port and gets proper medical aid.

The skipper planning a long cruise should determine if a potential crewperson has ever had duodenal ulcer or symptoms of duodenal ulcer, even though none was found on X-ray examination. The potential crewperson had best visit a doctor and discuss the symptom complex; hopefully a diagnosis can be established, the condition treated, and an emergency prevented.

ACUTE PERFORATION OF DUODENAL ULCER

A male with past history of recurrent abdominal pain or diagnosed duodenal ulcer awakes at 0400 hours groaning with pain. It doubles him
up; he feels cut in two through his upper abdomen. The pain gradually
spreads (an hour or two or three) over the entire abdomen. He retches,
but raises no vomit (see figure 32).

Examine him:

1. Apprehensive, sweating, pale, and in severe pain.
2. Pulse one hundred beats per minute or faster.
3. His abdomen is rigid, boardlike; if thumped, it sounds and feels
   like a wooden table.
4. His temperature (oral) is subnormal, but gradually elevates
   over the next twelve hours.

Treatment for suspected perforated ulcer:

1. Give him absolutely nothing by mouth.
2. Administer Demerol 75–100 mg by injection soon and every
   four hours as necessary for pain.
3. Pass nasogastric tube, continuously siphon or bulb suction to
   keep his stomach empty.
4. Log fluid intake and output as for acute appendicitis.
5. Supply daily parenteral fluids as for acute appendicitis. By injection, give Rocephin 1 to 2 grams daily, depending on the size
   of the patient and the severity of the illness (see package insert
   for this medicine).
6. If the patient has difficulty voiding, pass a catheter and leave
   in-lying. This probably will not be necessary.
7. Keep the patient in his bunk.

Follow-up care of perforated ulcers may be necessary for five to ten
days or even longer:

1. Keep the patient bunk-fast, control pain, and supply parenteral
   fluids and antibiotics until:
   a. Nausea and pain subside,
   b. Oral temperature is normal,
   c. Abdominal tenderness and rigidity relent.
2. Stop antibiotics when oral temperature is normal for twenty-
   four hours.
3. When abdominal pain and nausea completely subside, clamp
   the stomach tube shut. If patient does not vomit in twelve
   hours, remove the tube. If he does vomit before this time, re-
   open the tube and continue the siphonage and drainage a bit

longer. After the tube is removed, start sips of water by mouth, gradually increasing to full bland diet, and resume program described for treatment of uncomplicated ulcer.

4. Allow the patient out of his bunk when all symptoms subside, when he is eating a bland diet and feels strong. It will be some time before he is able to resume any duties aboard ship.

Discussion of Perforated Duodenal Ulcer
Upon perforation, a hole in the duodenal wall replaces the ulcer. This defect allows the acid and alkaline secretions of the gut, plus ingested food and fluids, to leak into the peritoneal cavity. These digestive enzymes burn the peritoneal surfaces and produce a chemical peritonitis. The systemic effect on circulation and regular body metabolism is similar to that produced by heat burn on the body surface. Untreated, such peritonitis is a distinct threat to life.

The peritoneal cavity can defend itself from the single spill at the time of perforation provided that it stops promptly. Treatment aims to stop it: Nothing is taken by mouth and the nasogastric tube sucks out indigenous secretions as fast as they form.

The great omentum, a fold of peritoneum hung from the stomach, then swings over the perforation in the duodenum. It secretes a sticky exudate similar to that made by inflamed bowel loops after a ruptured appendix. In a few days this will seal off the hole. Meanwhile, you must sustain life with parenteral fluids and prevent infection with antibiotics.

BLEEDING DUODENAL ULCER

A twenty-six year-old sailor comes from the head, puzzled. He has just had a large, black, liquid bowel movement. "It looks gummy and black like tar," he says, "and I feel weak and dizzy."

Ask him:

1. "Have you ever had an ulcer before?"

He says, "Two years ago I had stomach pain, X rays proved negative for ulcer. My doctor gave me Zantac for three weeks and a bland diet and the pain stopped."

2. "Have you had any pain in your stomach lately?"
"No, I haven't."
3. Do you feel like vomiting?"
"Yes, a little bit."

Examine him:

1. He is pale and frightened-looking (even under a good suntan).
2. His pulse is 90 to 120 beats per minute.
3. His oral temperature is 98°F or subnormal, 97–98°F.
4. There is a tender spot on his abdomen, two inches above and two inches to the right of his belly button (see figure 31).
5. His lower abdomen gurgles and rumbles.

If more than two of the above symptoms are present, suspect a bleeding duodenal ulcer.

1. Put him to bed.
2. Give two ounces of milk every hour until 2300 hours daily.
3. Allow in addition only water or tea with sugar by mouth.
4. Give Rocephin 1 or 2 grams by injection (see package insert for further information on dosage).
5. Give Demerol 75 mg by injection, soon.
6. He may vomit dark "coffee-grounds" material. This may precede the black diarrhea. Emesis (vomiting) increases fright. Repeat Demerol 75 mg every four hours to control apprehension.
7. He may have one or several more liquid, black, foul-smelling stools.

The ulcer will usually stop bleeding after forty-eight hours with the above treatment.

1. Nausea and emesis subside.
2. Pulse is slower than 100 beats per minute.
3. Sweating is less or stops.
4. Apprehension lessens; stop Demerol.
5. Black diarrhea stops.

Follow-up treatment:

1. Keep the patient in bed.
2. Have him chew and swallow two tablets of Pepto-Bismol every two waking hours and at bedtime.
3. Begin feedings every four hours: milk (canned or powdered), soft or boiled eggs, mashed potatoes, rice, oatmeal, tapioca, macaroni and cheese, or any food that does not cause indigestion. Give as much as the patient wants.

The patient will improve over the next two to three days. If above diet is tolerated on the fourth or fifth day after onset of bleeding:

1. Start ulcer diet prescribed for an uncomplicated ulcer.
2. Discontinue the Rocephin and use Cipro 500 mg by mouth every 12 hours (see package insert).

3. The patient may have dark, but not liquid, stools for several days after other symptoms subside.
4. Give a Dulcolax rectal suppository if needed.
5. Allow the patient to resume activity gradually; he will be weak for several days to two weeks.
6. A patient whose bleeding ulcer fails to stop (i.e., black vomiting and diarrhea continue more than twenty-four hours) requires sophisticated medical care quickly. Holler for help! Call MAS if you are a subscriber. Continue treatment until help arrives.

Discussion—Bleeding Duodenal Ulcer
The duodenal ulcer bleeds when it erodes a sizable artery. This does not hurt much because a blood film shields the ulcer base from irritating duodenal contents. Blood in the gut produces dramatic symptoms. In the stomach hydrochloric acid converts it to acid hematin. This looks like old coffee grounds and is very nauseating. Violent hematemesis (vomiting of blood) follows.

In the lower intestine, to which it is propelled by the peristaltic motion of the bowels, the digestive ferments and bacteria turn blood into a black, gummy, foul-smelling bowel movement. This, too, is irritating and a tarry-stool diarrhea follows. A nasty by-product is a considerable amount of gas which can be heard gurgling in the lower abdomen.

Both the systemic response and conditions at the ulcer site combine to prolong bleeding: hemorrhage anywhere in the body incites a general alarm reaction—the adrenal glands secrete norepinephrine which accelerates the pulse, increases the heart output, and raises blood pressure; digestive enzymes, mainly hydrochloric acid at the ulcer site, repeatedly dissolve clots before they firmly plug the bleeding vessel.

Treatment is best done early, for continued severe bleeding depletes clotting mechanisms and induces a state of general circulatory insufficiency that depresses all defense mechanisms. If you cannot stop bleeding from a duodenal ulcer within twelve hours, you will need outside help because blood transfusions may be necessary.

In summary then, it is evident that a duodenal ulcer may heal without developing any complications if treated early and thoroughly with rest, diet, antibiotics, antacids, and Tagamet. Although managing the simple duodenal ulcer on shipboard is troublesome, it is much better than allowing it to go untreated. As a matter of fact, 80 to 95 percent of duodenal ulcers when treated do heal promptly, nowadays.

It is also true that abdominal pain is usually not serious. But watch it carefully always. Then the occasional case of appendicitis, gallbladder disease, or duodenal ulcer will be recognized for early treatment.

GENITOURINARY EMERGENCIES

One Wednesday, at 1300 hours, as you participate in an offshore sailing event, a two-pole spinnaker jibe is in progress, and one of the foredeck gang unwisely straddles a pole. The foreguy is freed, and a gust hoists the sail skyward. The wayward pole crunches his crotch and throws him half overboard. Pulled back aboard, he falls to the deck groaning and holding his smashed testicles.

1. Get him below. He will be weak and in a shocklike condition, sweating and pale, with a rapid pulse.
2. Put cold packs, ice if possible, on the injured parts. They will swell remarkably.
3. Give him Demerol 100–125 mg by injection, soon.
4. Raise the race escort vessel by radiotelephone. Indicate that you have a casualty who needs evacuation. The escort vessel reports she is 360 miles from your position. At 10 knots, they will rendezvous with you in approximately thirty-six hours.

By 2000 hours your patient's penis and testicles have swollen massively. He passes a few drops of bloody urine with considerable effort and pain.

At 2300 hours he complains not only of lower abdominal pain but of a marked desire to urinate plus the inability to pass more than a drop or two of bloody urine.

Break out the prepackaged urethral catheterization tray (see figure 33). Contents vary, but all brands contain:

1. A Foley self-retaining catheter, size 14–15 fr,
2. Plastic cups and antiseptic solution,
3. A graduated basin to measure urine,
4. Lubricant for the catheter.

The procedure is:

1. Medicate the patient for the pain and for the anxiety of the impending procedure with Demerol 75 mg and Valium 5 mg, both by injection 30 to 60 minutes before cathcterization.
2. Open the prepackaged urethral catheterization tray. Spread out the sterile towel and neatly dump the contents onto this.
3. Scrub your hands for ten minutes with Betadine and fresh water sterilized by boiling for twenty minutes.
4. Put on sterile gloves.
5. Pour the antiseptic solution into one of the plastic cups.
6. Have the patient lie flat on his back with his knees drawn up.

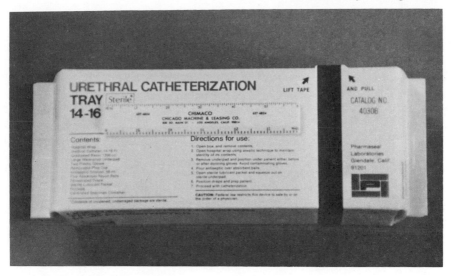

Fig. 33. Prepackaged urethral catheterization tray.

7. Elevate the tip of the patient's penis in left gloved fingers.
8. Wipe it well with antiseptic solution.
9. Lubricate the tip of the catheter. Insert it into the urinary meatus (the outlet in the penis) with the right hand.
10. Advance the catheter steadily. Have the patient take a series of deep breaths. Keep steady pressure on the catheter but do not jab it.
11. The catheter will pop into the bladder. Urine flow indicates the catheter is in place.
12. Tape the catheter to the leg, or if you have used a Foley self-retaining catheter, inflate the balloon (see figure 34).
13. Give Bactrim DS twice daily while the catheter is in place and for two days after its removal.
14. Urge oral fluids. Keep intake over 2500 cc (2 quarts) per day.

You have established urinary drainage and have begun antibiotics to prevent infection. There remains only the usual care of the bunk-fast patient and control of pain. Swelling and pain of penis and testicles should gradually subside. If the urine is red with blood at first, it will gradually clear.

It is an unlikely but possible event that

1. The patient is unable to void any urine at all. If the Foley catheter is in place and a good urine flow is not established, it is possible that blood clots in the urine are blocking the catheter.

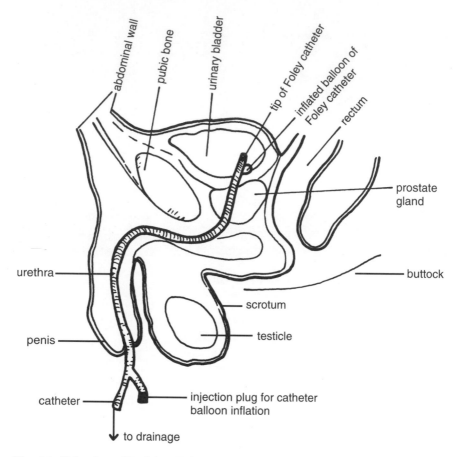

abdominal wall

pubic bone

urinary bladder

tip of Foley catheter

inflated balloon of
Foley catheter

rectum

prostate
gland

urethra

buttock

scrotum

testicle

penis

catheter

injection plug for catheter
balloon inflation

to drainage

Fig. 34. Side view of in-lying Foley catheter.

Irrigation of the catheter with sterile water or sterile salt solution may relieve the problem.

2. You are unable to pass a catheter.

The bladder will be distended and must be emptied. Complete urinary retention may be fatal in three to five days. Proceed as follows:

1. Gently percuss or feel the outline of the distended bladder. It is located in the lower abdomen immediately above the pubis bone (see figure 35).

2. Wash the abdominal wall over the distended bladder well with Betadine and sterile water. Shave the area and paint with antiseptic.

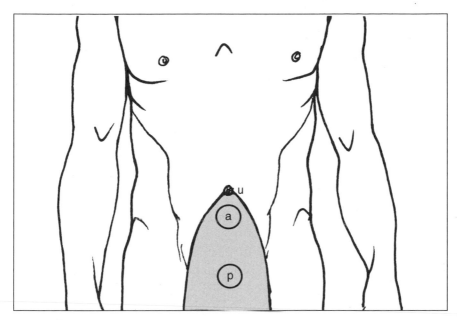

Fig. 35. Location of distended urinary bladder. Perform a cystotomy at (a), half-way between pubis (p) and umbilicus (u).

3. Wash your hands for ten minutes with Betadine and fresh sterile water. Put on sterile gloves.
4. Plunge a three-inch spinal No. 18 or other large hypodermic needle straight through the abdominal wall into the bladder. Urine flowing out will tell you when it is in place.
5. Remove as much urine as possible. Suck it out with a big syringe. If you do not have one, simply press on the abdominal wall alongside the needle, being careful not to dislodge it, and the urine will flow out.
6. When you have removed as much urine as possible, withdraw the needle swiftly and wipe the puncture wound with an antiseptic.
7. Repeat every one to two days until patient voids, catheterization is successful, or the patient is evacuated.

Discussion—Genitourinary Emergencies
The serious genitourinary emergency at sea is urinary retention—inability to pass water. The likely causes are:

1. Local injury to penis, scrotum, or perineum (crotch),

2. Reflex inhibition of urination due to nonlocal injury or severe illness,
3. Swelling of the prostate gland.

Direct injury may transect the urethra—the tube leading from the bladder, through the prostate gland and penis, to the outside (see figure 34). Swelling of the prostate gland or other surrounding tissues may squeeze it shut, even if it is intact.

Rupture of an artery may fill the bladder with big clots that plug the urethra. These will not obstruct passage of a catheter and may be removed by irrigation with sterile water.

Nervous impulses can inhibit voiding and produce reflex urinary retention even though no mechanical obstruction to the urinary tract exists. Urination by the healthy male demands complex sequential reactions. The start is voluntary; contraction of the urinary bladder which follows closely is involuntary. Control of the sphincter at the bladder outlet is partly voluntary (as when you hold your water through social necessity) and partly involuntary (once the stream is started, it is very difficult to close it off). Finally, the expelling of the last few drops of urine is voluntary. Certain healthy males always go to the end of the line at a public urinal. Nervous inhibition gives them a bashful bladder. Serious illness or injury that requires bed rest and sedation may lead to a similar inability to void.

It is always possible that the patient with reflex retention will void. The erect position may enable him to urinate; help him to stand beside his bunk.

Eventually the bladder will empty itself automatically. The agony of awaiting this may be more than either of you chooses to endure. But needle cystotomy is not usually indicated unless mechanical obstruction and/or traumatic division of the urethra is suspected.

Catheterize after twelve to eighteen hours of retention to relieve painful distension. Remove as much urine as possible. Afterwards withdraw the catheter, urge fluids, and he will probably be able to void spontaneously in a few hours.

If you have to catheterize him a second time, leave the catheter in place for three to four days. Give Bactrim DS, one twice daily for three days after a single catheter passage. Give the same dose of the same drug daily while the catheter is in-lying and for two days after its removal.

Prostatic infection as a cause of extrinsic urinary tract obstruction with retention is discussed in chapter 7, p. 102.

Benign (nonmalignant) enlargement of the prostate may produce retention in older men. The onset is gradual over a long period. The first symptom is nocturia—getting up at night to void—followed after some time by partial retention with frequent spillage of small amounts. Unless retention is complete do not pass a catheter; the individual will maintain satisfactory temporary drainage by frequent spilling (overflow) incontinence of small amounts of urine.

If retention becomes complete, then attempt catheterization. You may have difficulty. If you fail, you will have to do a needle cystotomy every one to two days until the patient is removed from your care. Use antibiotics as for other catheter procedures.

One final word about bladder infection (acute cystitis): It is much more common in women, who may or may not have fever, chills, and frequent, painful urination, but extremely rarely urinary retention. Bactrim DS taken twice a day for five days usually relieves the condition.

Should urinary retention occur, passage of a catheter in the female is much simpler than in the male. Her urethra is much shorter and less subject to obstruction. The only problem you encounter is finding the urethra. It is forward, just behind the clitoris.

CHAPTER 7

The Use of Antibiotics

On November 8 the 28-foot sloop *Wa* left Mahe, Seychelles Islands, starting on the second half of a circumnavigation. Aboard were Pete, Addie, and their cat, Coco. Mozambique Island—the next landfall—lay 1,500 miles south and west beyond a belt of calms, contrary winds, erratic currents, and generally miserable sailing. Five days later, still 400 miles away from Mozambique, a 40-knot gale blew up, dead on the nose.

At 0900 a huge wave swept the steering vane overboard. It dragged behind as *Wa* lifted and dropped on the 25-foot waves. Pete spent a frantic hour thrashing around on his abdomen over the tiny fantail to bring the damn thing back aboard.

At 1900 the wind dropped to 20 knots and hauled to the quarter. Pete and Addie started three-on and three-off watches to steer by hand in the confused and tumbling seas. Addie relieved Pete at 1200. He went aft to void but was unable to pass more than a few drops of dark urine that burned like fire. Shortly afterwards he had a shaking chill. His oral temperature was 102°F.

Pete drank as much water as he could for the next three hours but still was unable to pass more than a few drops of urine at a time, although he had a growing urge to void. Dull throbbing pain grew more intense at the base of his scrotum and radiated into the small of his back.

He managed to stand his next watch from 1600 to 2000, but felt "a little fuzzy" during the last hour. Addie stood by to prevent a flying jibe.

By 2100, the urge to urinate generated a massive ache through his lower abdomen, and down the inside of both thighs. His teeth chattered with pain and fever. Still he could not void.

So Pete held the tiller while Addie went below and broke out the presterilized catheterization set. She took over the helm and Peter catheterized himself (technique described in chapter 6, pp. 97–98).

The process, he reported, was "mighty uncomfortable," but the relief, after he had drained away nearly a quart of dark, cloudy urine, was "worth it."

When the catheter was placed in his bladder, he inflated the balloon (see figure 34) and left it there since he was not sure that he could void and the passage of the catheter that one time was all he wanted to undergo.

At 0200, he unclamped the catheter and drained a pint of dark urine. He had another chill. His temperature was 101.2°F. The pain of urinary retention was relieved but he still had considerable discomfort at the base of the scrotum and down the inside of both thighs.

He had a urinary tract infection, probably related to irregular eating and drinking, exposure, and the local trauma inflicted as he lay extended over the cockpit trying to salvage the steering vane. This urinary tract infection swelled the prostate gland, which in turn shut off his ability to void.

To treat this, he took one tablet Bactrim DS at 0200, one more at 0800, and then one every twelve hours for the next five days. He drank two large glasses of water with each dose of the pills.

By 1000, 13 November, his pain was relieved. His temperature was 99°F and he had lost the "fuzzy" feeling.

Wisely, however, he continued to take Bactrim DS twice a day for a total of ten days of treatment and to drink two glasses of water with each dose. By November 15, he had no distress. On this day he removed the catheter and was able to void readily with only a light residual burning. Had he not responded to Bactrim DS after several days it would have been wise to switch to Cipro 500 mg three times daily. There are times when the usual medications just don't work as anticipated.

Exposure, irregular voiding, dehydration due to poor eating and drinking conditions, plus the knocking about on a small (or large) boat may produce urinary tract infections. As in this case, the prostate gland may swell and cut off urine flow. Catheterization prevents severe and possibly fatal complications.

Urinary tract infections are common in women, too. However, rarely do they cause urinary retention because the female urinary tract from the bladder to the outside world is very short and there are no structures about it which can swell and close it off.

Pete's diagnosis was based upon fever above 101°F, which suggested infection, and the symptoms relating to the genitourinary system which localized this infection.

PNEUMONIA

After five months visiting in Nuku Hiva, Pete and Addie left for Penrhyn, about 1,100 miles to the west. The wind vane was repaired and there was no need to keep watches. Nonetheless, at 0530 on 2 May, Addie got drenched by a sudden shower because she was meditating while watching the tropical sunrise. She finished her watch, but she was shivering and uncomfortable when Pete relieved her at 0800.

She came on watch again at 1200, but felt miserable, "ached all over," and her throat hurt. She stood the watch but about halfway through she began to cough and her chest hurt when she did so. Her temperature was 100°F.

At 1500 she was resting in her bunk and had a shaking chill. The cough became worse and she produced some yellow sputum. She felt short of breath and when she tried to take a deep breath her left ribs hurt. Her temperature at this time was 103°F. Pete noted that her nostrils flared with her rapid breathing, twenty-eight times a minute, whereas normal resting breathing is sixteen to eighteen times a minute. Addie had pneumonia.

Formerly penicillin would have been the drug of choice. Today, however, about 25% of the strains of the usual bacteria causing pneumonia in the U.S.A. are resistant to penicillin, and the resistance rate is far higher in many distance counties so it would be best to use an alternative medicine such as Keflex 500 mg tablets, four times a day.

Twelve hours later Addie's temperature was 99°F and she felt much better. She was well enough to stand her watch. Addie protested that she felt fine and didn't take the Keflex. She would have been wiser to do so.

Twelve hours later she had another chill and her temperature following this was 104°F. All symptoms returned. Keflex was restarted.

By May 4, her temperature was 100°F at 0800 hours and 103.6°F at 1600 hours. She felt weak, was breathing fast, and her cough hurt more.

On May 5 she was about the same or worse.

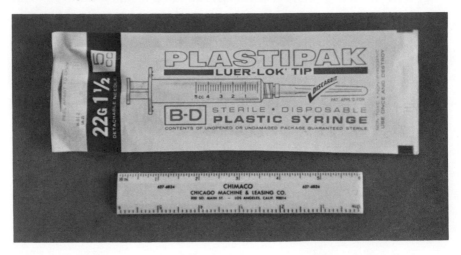

Fig. 36. Prepackaged sterile syringe and needle.

On May 6 she felt no better. Since she was not responding to the Keflex, it was discontinued and she was given Cipro 500 mg three times a day. Remember antibiotic therapy is tricky and without laboratory assistance making changes in medicines can be a difficult decision.

On May 7 her temperature was again normal and she felt much stronger, although she still had a cough which was productive. Pete continued the same medicine and by the third day she felt well again, although she was somewhat weak.

Her temperature remained normal and this time Addie stayed well until they arrived at the Kiribati islands.

RULES FOR USE OF ANTIBIOTICS

Pete is not a physician. However, his management of these two serious infections they encountered illustrates the basic rules for treatment of infectious diseases with antibiotic drugs. Simply stated, the rules are:

1. Use antibiotics only for serious infections.
2. Select the antibiotic that will be most likely to kill the attacking bacterium (see figure 37). In the real world the physician uses clinical judgment based upon experience, subtle physical findings, and laboratory guidance. In this setting you will be making an educated guess at best.
3. When you select the proper drug, be sure the patient is not allergic to it. Ask the patient; he or she will probably know. If the patient is allergic to it, you must use another drug.
4. Give the suggested dose at the proper intervals. Expect improvement (lowered fever, patient feeling better) within twenty-four to thirty-six hours.
5. After the patient's temperature is normal, continue the same dose at the same intervals for forty-eight hours longer.
6. For mild infections five days of antibiotic treatment might be sufficient; in this setting, however, it might be better to treat all infections as if they were severe and continue the antibiotics for seven days. In any case, the antibiotics should not be discontinued until the patient is doing much better and is fever-free for forty-eight hours.
7. If there is no improvement in the patient's condition within a week, one should consider trying a different antibiotic, starting with the larger dose specified in the package insert for the new antibiotic while continuing to give the old antibiotic for the first twenty-four hours.

The Use of Antibiotics

Fever 102° F+ with or without chills

Local symptoms	Likely disease	Treatment
Cough, chest pain, labored breathing, yellow sputum	bronchitis or pneumonia	Keflex 500 mg one or two tablets four times a day or Cipro 500 mg two or three times a day for seven days.
Earache—pain when earlobe pulled down	otitis media (middle ear infection)	Same as pneumonia.
Sore throat—hurts to swallow. Throat fiery red, may have yellow spots on tonsils	strep sore throat	Same as pneumonia.
Frequent and burning urination; urgency	cystitis	Bactrim DS one tablet every twelve hours until symptom-free for forty-eight hours. Take for a minimum of five days—preferably seven.
Symptoms of cystitis (above) plus pain in back and tenderness between lowest rib and spine	pyelonephritis (kidney infection)	Bactrim DS one tablet every twelve hours for ten days.
Swollen testicles; pain at base of scrotum	epididymitis or prostatitis	Cipro 500 mg two times a day for seven days.
Discharge from penis without fever; exposure	gonorrhea or chlamydia	Cipro 500 mg one dose only accompanied by Doxycycline 100 mg two times a day for two weeks.

Fig. 37. Antibiotic selection chart for common infections. For drug dosage for children, see chapter 17. For severe infections, note the larger doses recommended in the package inserts.

8. Failure of a patient to improve after a week on the second antibiotic indicates that a more serious problem than anticipated may be present. A radio consultation with a physician is now imperative. Then reduce antibiotic drug dose to one-half the amount, given at the same intervals as before, for another twenty-four hours.

Before administering any antibiotic, it is wise to review the package insert with the medication you wish to use. It will confirm you are doing the correct thing, advise on what to anticipate, and warn of dangers.

Many diseases that produce high fever are not responsive to antibiotics, so after a reasonable trial as outlined above, stop antibiotics.

Use the chart (see figure 37) to help select the most likely antibiotic as given in rule 2. If the patient has a high fever and symptoms are indefinite or you cannot decide, do try an antibiotic. The chart is only a rough and ready rule of thumb to help you in your selection. Try it on your own if the chart does not answer your specific questions.

Remember, too, that most infections you encounter will never be severe enough to require antibiotic treatment. Common colds are not responsive; most diarrheas are mild, of virus origin, and require only Pepto-Bismol, one teaspoonful after each loose stool (Pepto-Bismol also comes in tablets, with explicit directions for dosage on the box), or Lomotil and light diet for a few days. The other mild infections you will see will subside after a day or two of rest and light diet. Save the antibiotics for the severe infections.

Blood poisoning is discussed in chapter 3 on the follow-up care of wounds.

Discussion

Follow these rules to use the antibiotic drugs to best advantage. A physician shoreside with a laboratory available might take a culture of the infecting bug and test it for sensitivity to various antibiotics before he or she starts treatment. However, this takes a day or two and often the physician will begin treatment with the drug of his or her choice simultaneously. Pediatricians do this often because infections progress rapidly in children; veterinarians usually do it, too.

At sea you gauge successful treatment by the patient's response. A fever thermometer measures this best. You should take several in metal cases. Body temperature stays constant in a healthy person with about a 1° daily variation that relates to activity. Highest daily temperature is usually at 1600–1800 hours and lowest at 0300–0400 hours. This explains why the midwatch is such a bore. Not only are you chilly and alone while the rest of the world sleeps warm and comfortable below, but your body temperature is at its lowest ebb.

How does heat regulation relate to a person with an infection? Systemic infections constrict the surface blood vessels and drive blood into the deeper tissues where heat loss is diminished.

The infected person first feels his skin cold; he has a chill. Heat production continues and body temperature rises. Shortly a new balance between heat production and heat loss is established at a higher temperature.

Now the patient feels warm all over; he has a fever. It is nature's way of responding to infection. The elevated temperature accelerates antibacterial antibody production.

Severe systemic infections that require antibiotic treatment may develop quickly or slowly. It was obvious that Addie, who developed shaking chills, a fever of 103°F in a few hours, together with chest pain and a cough producing yellow sputum, had severe bronchitis and/or pneumonia. Keflex in standard doses was given quickly.

Recurrence of her pneumonia shows the error of stopping treatment too soon. A few hardy germs still lived in her lungs and renewed the attack. It was necessary to add another antibiotic (Cipro) to the Keflex to overcome this new growth of resistant germs.

It is less dramatic when such a fever builds up to this level over two or three days. However, a fever of 103° F on two successive days, even if it develops gradually, warrants a trial of antibiotic treatment.

You will need more than one antibiotic and more than one form of certain ones to cover the effective range of antibacterial treatment.

Rocephin is a potent broad-spectrum antibiotic drug for intramuscular or intravenous administration. When severe nausea and/or vomiting preclude the use of oral antibiotics this will be the drug of choice. When the patient has resumed normal gastrointestinal function, you may switch to the oral antibiotic suggested.

The usual adult dose of Rocephin is 1–2 grams daily. With severe infections use 2 grams every twelve hours. For pediatric patients the once a day total dose is 50–75 mg/kg of body weight. The total dose in severe pediatric cases should not exceed 2 grams a day.

There is a sufficient range of strong antibiotics recommended for your first aid kit. It cannot be stressed enough that if your patient does not respond in several days, you should switch to an alternative medicine. As always, radio consultation with a physician is preferred.

Certain other infectious diseases produce almost no fever and yet are best treated with antibiotics. One should try to exclude allergies as a cause for the illness, but with a patient exhibiting persistent and significant symptoms, antibiotics may be tried.

SEXUALLY TRANSMITTED DISEASES (STD)

You are four or five days out to sea from San Francisco towards Tahiti and your port watch captain shows up one morning with a shameful face, a penile discharge, and a complaint of great distress when urinating.

His last night in San Francisco he went "out on the town." Examine his penis. Have him squeeze the urethra; pus oozes forth. The diagnosis may be gonorrhea or chlamydia. This must be treated and, since he may have also contracted syphilis on the same visit, the treatment must be extended to cover multiple STDs.

1. Give one dose of Cipro 500 mg by mouth.
2. Give Doxycycline 100 mg two times a day for fourteen days. Hopefully this strong and prolonged dose of medicine will cure syphilis that might have been acquired at the same encounter.

(Penicillin injections for syphilis treatment over this several week period could be very difficult. Also gonorrhea is usually resistant to even very high doses of penicillin therapy.)

3. After this treatment, advise him most strongly to have a blood test for syphilis in three to six months, a check for the AIDS antigen, and further studies if he has continuing urethral problems.

If your port watch captain is a female, her complaints may be few or multiple, including pelvic and/or abdominal pain, vaginal discharge, frequent urination or burning upon urination, and urethral discharge. She may have a fever. Doing a pelvic examination could be very helpful, but without medical experience in this area, it is best avoided. As in the case of the male patient, if the female has these symptoms some days after having intercourse without using a condom and with a new partner, it would strongly suggest a diagnosis of sexually transmitted disease. The treatment would be the same as that for a male patient.

DRUG SENSITIVITY

Allergic and sensitivity reactions may appear after any drug administration. You will avoid serious problems by asking the patient if she is sensitive before you give her a drug. Usually she will know. If she is or if there is any doubt, do not give it to her—you might kill her.

Immediate drug reaction, called anaphylactic shock, is dramatic and frightening. Shortly after the administration (most often by injection) of a drug, the patient turns pale, collapses, and becomes pulseless. She may be conscious or unconscious. Apnea may occur.

1. Give mouth-to-mouth resuscitation if needed.
2. Give adrenaline .5 cc of 1/1000 by injection. Give half of the dose near the site at which the first drug was injected and the other half in another area.
3. Keep the patient warm, maintain her in a level or slightly head-down position.
4. After she begins to recover—color returns, pulse is again palpable, sweating stops—give stimulants such as coffee or tea.
5. If she does not begin to recover within five to ten minutes, give an additional .5 cc of 1/1000 adrenaline by injection.
6. After recovery, keep her in her bunk for twelve hours.

It is advisable to have ampules of adrenaline readily available with a syringe for administration whenever potent drugs (antibiotics, etc.) are given.

Delayed drug sensitivity reactions are less awesome although their appearance means all drugs must be stopped except adrenaline and antihistamines such as Benadryl.

Hives are raised, reddish-white welts that appear over the body surface and indicate allergy to a drug. They are chiefly annoying because they itch.

1. Stop all drugs.
2. Give antihistamines such as Benadryl 25 mg every four to six hours or Claritin 10 mg daily.

Skin rashes also signal drug sensitivity and appear as reddish blotches starting usually on the abdomen and spreading over the whole body. These require the same measures as hives.

Nausea and diarrhea may occur with gastrointestinal allergy to some drugs.

1. Stop the drug.
2. Use Phenergan 25 mg suppositories every eight hours until nausea is controlled.
3. If diarrhea is a problem, give two Lomotil tablets immediately and one after each subsequent movement until stools are normal. Give no more than eight pills in a twenty-four-hour period.

If any drug sensitivity reaction, anaphylactic shock, hives, skin rashes, or gastrointestinal upsets occur and you have given by injection a long-acting drug, the reaction may continue for some time. After partial recovery, be on the lookout for a recurrence of symptoms and treat it again.

SKIN PROBLEMS

Skin diseases rarely threaten life but they can make it nearly unendurable, particularly in the tropics. At the specific request of the skipper of the *Wa,* whose crew suffered much in this way, a few notes on skin diseases are included here.

The exotic jungle rot fungus and fearsome boils observed in the tropics are essentially the same athlete's foot (dermatophytosis) and staphylococcus skin infections seen in all climates. The constant moisture and warmth make them grow luxuriantly like all other tropical flora and fauna. Sores become infected easily and heal poorly for this reason; athlete's foot rages wildly beyond the confines of the toes.

Lack of cleanliness also encourages infection, both fungal and bacterial. The first principle then is to keep the skin clean and dry and as free of salt as possible. Wipe the exposed parts at least daily with a small amount of fresh water. Avoid sunburn, windburn, and maceration of skin from prolonged exposure to salt water.

When fungus infection develops, expect it not only between the toes and in the crotch but in the underarm and in open sores anywhere on the body. Daily application of 1% Silvadene salve on all affected areas will help heal sores but more slowly than is common in temperate climates. Exposure and drying also help to clear fungus.

Boils and furuncles should be treated with daily antibacterial ointment application and systemic antibiotics such as Keflex 500 mg four times a day or Cipro 500 mg twice daily. Skin irritations and rashes that produce severe, maddening itching can be controlled by daily application of a cream or ointment containing hydrocortisone.

Resistant ulcers are treated with antibacterial drugs. Adequate oral intake of Vitamins A, C, and perhaps D will encourage healing of skin lesions. A and D ointment helps to heal resistant sores due to exposure, drying, and salt encrustation.

Management of wound infections is discussed in chapter 3.

A 1% hydrocortisone cream is extremely efficacious for allergic or irritated skin conditions. Unless the skin area is infected, there is relatively little concern about using this daily until the disorder clears.

CHAPTER 8

The Unconscious Patient

Force-Eight weather catches you somewhere between Newport News and Barbados. Your yawl, *Restless,* running under jib and jigger, bangs into a sizable wave and tosses the navigator headfirst into a bulkhead. He quivers, then silently rolls to and fro across the deck.

1. Be sure he is breathing. Resuscitate him if he is not.

A complete examination (see chapter 1) shows the following:

2. A large lump on the top of his head.
3. No response to questions; thumb pressure on the eyebrow elicits a groan—he doesn't brush your thumb away.
4. Pupils of both eyes are dilated widely and do not contract when a strong light is shone directly into them.
5. His arms and legs are flaccid—lift them and let go; they flop back to the deck.
6. The remainder of your examination finds no injury.

The navigator has a severe head injury. You will have to try to keep him alive until his brain recovers. This is the order of priority.

1. Maintain an open airway.
   a. Keep his head a foot lower than his body. If he vomits, then he won't aspirate the material into his lungs and drown.
   b. Use a bulb syringe, a rag, or your finger to clear mucus, vomit, or his tongue out of the airway. This is a 24-hour-a-day responsibility. Post a continuous watch.
2. Provide adequate parenteral fluids (salt solution) according to chapters 4 and 6. The basic daily requirement is 1000 cc, not 1500 cc as for other conditions.
3. Insert a Foley catheter as he will be incontinent and you will need to measure his urinary output. Give Rocephin 1 gram daily prophylactically.

4. If there is fever over 100°F, persistent bleeding, or clear fluid draining from the nose or either ear, increase the Rocephin injection to 2 grams daily.
5. Lash him securely in his bunk. Loosen ties; turn him over, and relash every few hours.
6. Log daily at 1200 and 2400 hours:
   a. State of consciousness: comatose, drowsy, agitated, alert.
   b. Reflexes: pupil response to light, cough, swallowing (elicit by pressure on Adam's apple), response to pressure on the eyebrow (Does he groan and attempt to push your thumb away?).
   c. Rectal temperature and respirations per minute.
   d. Spontaneous, purposeful movements of extremities: yes or no.

He may recover in hours or days. Your log anticipates this:

1. Reflexes return. Pupils contract to strong light. Gag reflex returns—touch soft palate with tongue blade or spoon handle. Cough present—blow smoke in his face. He swallows when you press on his Adam's apple. Respiration is regular.
2. Purposeful movements start. He pushes your thumb away when you apply painful pressure to his eyebrow.
3. Regains consciousness—answers questions. Recovery may be incomplete—he may drift back and forth between consciousness and unconsciousness for a time.

Amnesia for the accident and a preceding period may persist; space and time orientation may be poor at first. It is safe to let him eat and drink when gag and cough reflexes are active. Or, he may remain comatose until you make port. In this case, you must keep up your supportive treatment.

Prolonged coma brings certain changes:

1. Increased amounts of mucus plug the airway. Insert a resuscitating tube—push a catheter through it and suck trachea and pharynx dry as often as needed; use a bulb syringe, a reversed air compressor, or your own lips.
2. Constipation can cause fecal impaction, bowel obstruction, and abdominal distension. Insert a Dulcolax rectal suppository every three days to prevent this.
3. Flaccid (paralyzed) arms and legs gradually become spastic and rigid. This makes turning the patient difficult, but he must be turned every four hours to prevent bedsores.

4. If coma persists more than four days: Pass a nasogastric tube for feeding and medication. If gag reflex is absent, this will be easy.

   a. After the tube is in place, bubble test it. Hold the outer end under water; if it bubbles, the inner end is in the lung. Remove the tube and reinsert so it no longer makes bubbles when the outer end is submerged.

   b. Squirt sugar water slowly (2 tbsp. sugar dissolved in a quart of water), two ounces every two hours from 0800 hours to 2400 hours daily into the tube. Clamp or tie it off between feedings.

   c. If step 2 is tolerated, add milk, eggs, mashed potatoes—any food that can be liquefied and passed through the tube.

   d. Note: If the patient retches or vomits at any time, get his head low, suck out the airway, and empty the stomach through the nasogastric tube.

   e. Check the tube (bubble test) before each and every feeding.

   f. Give antibiotic medication with tube feedings or use injectable antibiotics.

   g. Less parenteral fluids are needed when tube feedings start. Stop parenteral fluid injections when tube feedings produce 500 cc of urine in twenty-four hours. See chapter 21 for child's urine output.

   h. Wash mouth out daily with toothpaste, mouthwash, lemon juice, or Vitamin C tablets dissolved in water.

Patient's condition may deteriorate. Early, this is due to primary brain injury. Later, it may be due to continued bleeding into the brain, infection of the brain, pneumonia, urine retention, or bladder infection.

1. Periods of restlessness, irrational behavior at times alternating with coma, or a steadily deepening coma indicate further brain damage. Rising rectal temperature, 103°–106°F, also indicates complications.

2. Irregular breathing—periods of rapid, deep breathing alternating with periods of complete apnea (Cheyne-Stokes respiration)—indicates severe brain damage.

3. Shallow, rapid respiration with flaring nostrils and cough suggest pneumonia.

4. Cloudy urine may mean bladder infection. Pus extrudes from the urethral meatus about the catheter after it is in-lying a day or two. This is no reason to remove the catheter. Wipe away the discharge with antiseptic solution as needed.

5. Plug-up of the bladder catheter may occur.

6. Dilation of one pupil that fails to contract to light suggests severe damage to the opposite side of the brain. Bilateral persistently dilated pupils that do not contract to strong light indicate severe bilateral brain damage.

You cannot accurately assess the original or continuing brain damage or diagnose certainly which complications are developing. So you must treat all shotgun-like if your log shows the patient is worse.

1. Check airway; be sure it is clear.
2. Irrigate the urinary catheter; be sure it flows freely to and fro.
3. Double the dose of antibiotic or add a second drug (see chapter 7).
4. Give Decadron 4 mg (1 cc) by intramuscular injection every six hours for three injections.
5. For restlessness or delirium (difficult behavior to control) give Valium 10 mg by injection, no more often than every twelve hours. See chapter 18 for child's dose, or compute by Young's Rule.
6. Maintain necessary restraints to keep the patient from hurting himself.
7. For rising temperature (above 105°–106°F rectally), remove all clothing and bedding. Give repeated alcohol or cold-water sponge baths.

Two other conditions may follow a blow on the head, both dangerous but fortunately rare.

A middle meningeal artery syndrome follows a severe blow on the side of the head. There is usually a brief period of unconsciousness followed by apparent recovery. However, over the next few hours, the individual becomes confused, complains of severe headache, loses consciousness, develops deepening coma, and usually expires.

The blow has fractured the skull and torn the middle meningeal artery which lies under the bone. Continued arterial bleeding produces increasing pressure which leads to death.

Diagnosis can be suspected if one pupil dilates while the opposite one contracts to strong light. Treatment consists of boring a hole in the skull (trephination) to let the blood out and relieve the pressure.

Subdural hematoma, a syndrome produced by tearing of one of the veins in the meninges (the membranes surrounding the brain), is even more subtle. The original injury is often so slight that it is forgotten. Weeks or even months later, headache develops, followed by irrational behavior and finally, if untreated, coma and death.

Treatment for this condition is trephination (cutting a hole in the skull), requiring hospital neurosurgical care.

Discussion—Head Injury

In addition to head injury, diabetic coma, insulin shock, uremic poisoning, drug overdose, cerebrovascular accident (stroke or brain hemorrhage), or prolonged anoxia (as in near drowning) may produce coma.

Head injury is the most likely cause you will encounter. The unconscious patient is more helpless than a newborn babe whose squall at least attracts attention to discomfort or danger.

Successful treatment of coma demands vigilance and initiative. Do not despair; patients have completely recovered after twenty-nine days of profound unconsciousness.

A blow on the head (or jaw) may stop all brain function briefly. Joe Louis's boxing opponents learned this the hard way. For a minimum of ten seconds they were "out."

Vital functions—breathing, heartbeat, temperature control—returns in seconds; voluntary protective movements, in seconds to minutes; consciousness and coherent thought, in minutes to hours or sometimes days.

Concussion is poorly understood. The brain appears essentially unchanged to the naked eye, but new microscopic research indicates structural damage that may never heal. Complete interruption of service occurs while circuits appear normal. If concussion is the only injury to the brain, consciousness returns in a few minutes. A headache may persist for one to three weeks. Rest and Tylenol, or Tylenol #3, will control this. Aspirin should be avoided as it could increase bleeding. In addition to general concussion, a harder blow may cause local damage to brain tissue on the side struck or contra-coup, the opposite side, where transmitted force has banged the brain against the skull. A brain bruise forms like a hidden black eye. It differs from a real black eye in that the skull sharply limits swelling. Instead, the brain presses against bone, raises the pressure within the cranium (intracranial pressure), and squeezes blood out of its own tissue.

Various regions of the brain differ in their sensitivity to lack of oxygen. First to quit working is the cerebellum—controlling the thinking and voluntary movement centers. Increasing cerebral anoxia produces first irrational behavior, then semiconsciousness (patient asleep but can be aroused), finally deep coma, during which no purposeful movements take place even to remove painful stimulation (thumb pressed hard on an eyebrow), and patient cannot be roused.

The vital brain stem centers (at the base of the brain) that control breathing, circulation, and body temperature are more resistant to anoxia. They go about their daily tasks, albeit sometimes fitfully, with an oxygen supply that will not keep the sleeping cerebral cells awake. Failure of these centers indicates severe brain damage.

The respiratory center, in the brain stem, has two chemical controls. Most sensitive is its response to small increases in carbon dioxide in the arterial blood. When you walk a little faster, your muscles make a bit more carbon dioxide. Within seconds this circulates to the respiratory control center, which makes you breathe harder and blow off the excess carbon dioxide; slow down and within seconds your breathing is back to the normal rate for walking.

The second control—response to lowered oxygen content in arterial blood—is far less sensitive. Violent exercise (running the quarter-mile) demands so much oxygen for muscle function that the lungs cannot keep up the supply; it also produces more carbon dioxide than can be readily blown away. An oxygen debt and carbon dioxide excess results which you pay back by panting for several minutes after you stop running.

Anoxia following head injury decreases the sensitivity of the respiratory control center to carbon dioxide. Apnea stops respiratory exchange in the lungs. Carbon dioxide content of the blood rises, but the depressed respiratory center will not respond and oxygen content decreases; finally the combination overcomes the sleepy respiratory center. An oxygen debt and carbon dioxide excess, very like that following violent exercise, now make the unconscious patient pant. Shortly carbon dioxide drops and oxygen rises to normal levels. Apnea again develops. The cycle goes on. This is Cheyne-Stokes respiration—an eponym for those physicians who first described it. It is a very grave prognostic sign following head injury.

The center for circulation control, located also in the brain stem, responds more favorably to increased intracranial pressure following brain injury. It slows the heart rate (greater filling occurs between beats), stroke volume rises and increases systemic blood pressure in an effort to force more blood into the crowded, gasping brain cells.

The temperature control center is resistant to anoxia so marked changes in body temperature denote severe brain injury. Heat loss mechanisms (see chapter 5) fail; the temperature rises rapidly. If the center does not recover, body temperature of 107–108°F may cause irreparable brain damage.

The severity of the original injury will determine the degree of increased intracranial pressure and brain dysfunction. If the injury is not too great and if you support the vital functions, eventually brain swelling subsides, the neurons heal, consciousness returns, and gradual recovery follows.

The treatment outlined is supportive except for three specific measures: first, Decadron is an adrenal cortical hormone that reduces brain swelling directly; second, alcohol sponge baths reduce rising body temperature and protect the brain from heat damage until the temperature control center recovers; and third, the antibiotics control infection when blood will not clot, or clear fluid drains from the nose or the ear. Such liquid is cerebrospinal fluid formed in the brain. Its leaking denotes a fracture through the base of the skull. Unless prevented by antibiotics, bacteria may ascend through the cracked bone and infect the brain.

We have said little about fracture of the skull here. You cannot detect its location without an X ray and, except for the rare depressed fracture, it is of no immediate importance in emergency management at sea. It is damage to the brain that counts. To my knowledge, there is no tale of a skull that failed to knit if the brain beneath survived.

In summary, if you support brain stem centers that keep respiration, circulation, and temperature control working, you will keep the unconscious patient alive; however, this care is very difficult aboard. Early evacuation of the patient is mandatory.

You treat a patient with a spinal fracture and injury to the cord in much the same fashion. Depending upon the level of injury the victim will be paralyzed from the neck down (quadriplegic) or from the waist down (paraplegic). In a cervical fracture, he or she may be unconscious. This is rare in lower spinal injury. Your treatment will be to supply what you can of those functions that the patient cannot do. He or she may have to be fed, have an airway maintained, be given extra fluids, and may require an in-lying catheter just as an unconscious patient does. He or she will guide you in what is needed.

DELIRIUM AND OTHER BEHAVIOR PROBLEMS

On November 6, 1968, *Diastole,* a 36-foot cutter, headed south out of Los Angeles Harbor on the Mazatlan race. Her crew of six included Dr. Arthur Stritch as her physician-captain-navigator and five others.

Los Angeles was in the midst of an epidemic of Hong Kong flu and poor *Diastole*'s crew took the brunt. The weather was fair but she was sailed shorthanded. Dr. Stritch got the flu twenty-four hours out of port. Two days later, when he had recovered sufficiently to stagger into the cockpit and hold the wheel in a brave simulation of watch standing, two other members were flat on their bunks. And so it went.

Some 700 miles downwind, the midwatch got a squall; the spinnaker filled and *Diastole* began to run. The watch, two of the walking ill, saw the youngest crew member crawling up out of his bunk to the stern pulpit.

Suddenly there was a wild burst of screaming and singing audible even above the whistle of the wind. Dr. Stritch turned a flashlight aft. Balanced on one foot, holding to the backstay with one hand and gyrating back and forth, stark-naked and yelling at the top of his lungs, was the youngest member.

With no hope of reasoning with him, Dr. Art jumped up and grabbed the lad as he went wheeling off to port with the ship's roll. After a struggle, he was safe in the cockpit. Or was he? He kept jumping up, eyes rolling wildly. He was in his own private shrieking world; contact was impossible.

The others awakened. They wrestled him below, wiped him dry, and wrapped him in a blanket. He threw it off and started topside the moment they let go of his hands and feet. They managed to take a rectal temperature (one man sailed the boat while four accomplished this medical maneuver). It was 107°F. He had the "flu."

Dr. Stritch:

1. Wrapped him firmly in a blanket.
2. Had two crewmen hold him down.
3. Gave him by intravenous injection slowly over several minutes possibly up to 10 mg of Valium. (Intramuscular would have been just as effective. It would have been some minutes longer taking effect, however.)
4. Gave him aspirin 600 mg every four hours until his fever was down to 99° for twenty-four hours. Aspirin should be avoided in children with "flu" as it may increase the risk for Reye's syndrome, a very rare viral disorder involving the brain and liver.

Twenty minutes later the patient was snoring away as though fever, delirium, and irrational behavior on a small sailboat in the middle of a squall had never happened.

The next morning his temperature was somewhat lower. He had no further bouts of delirium—and he did not remember his midnight episode. Antibiotics are of no value in "flu"—it is a viral infection—except when there is secondary bacterial infection present. If the patient's recovery is slow or new symptoms arise, it might be wise to start him on Keflex 500 mg four times a day or Cipro 500 mg two times a day.

Discussion

Irrational, uncontrolled behavior is somewhat analogous to scrambling of electrical circuits. The elements of proper perception of various stimuli and relevant action are lost. Many times stimuli arising from such short circuits project outward sensory impressions which do not really exist (hallucinations).

Anoxia commonly will disorganize the brain patterns of reception and response. This is most likely due to loss of cerebral (controlling) function while the motor centers are still relatively intact. Such anoxia may result from high fever which demands so much oxygen for the body that it is in short supply in the brain. Or high temperatures may directly disorganize the brain cells themselves.

Drugs of various types will alter cerebral and brain stem function. And at times, withdrawal of drugs (or alcohol) may do the same.

Regardless of the cause, unruly behavior that endangers a person must be controlled. In the case described, had the boy not been restrained there is little doubt he would have been lost overboard. Many times moderate physical restraints will suffice. If some obvious cause for anoxia (a semiconscious patient with a partially obstructed airway) can be found and corrected, this may render the individual tractable. If it is necessary or evident from the outset that drug control is needed, Valium is the drug of choice—probably by injection, although it is possible that patients suffering a mild degree of troubled behavior can be talked into taking it by mouth.

Since the brain is already injured, these drugs should be used cautiously. Start with small doses (2½–5 mg Valium) and watch for half to three-quarters of an hour. Then you will not wind up with a patient who is too depressed to breathe and needs resuscitation.

Do not be afraid. Proceed slowly but do continue until you get the desired effect, i.e., a calm, tractable, or sleeping patient. There is really in the last analysis no dose of a drug, only the amount which produces the desired effect.

Head injury and delirium tremens from alcohol overindulgence are indications for extreme caution in the use of potent tranquilizers. But use them if you must.

Once you gain control, maintain it. Perhaps the cause will pass quickly as it did for the boy with the flu. Watch your patient carefully—the drug will not wear off all at once. You may note signs that suggest you had better repeat the dose after one or two or several hours. Stay ahead of your patient by careful observation.

Chronic anxiety and depressive states that develop on long cruises are beyond the scope of this book. They may cause unpleasantness aboard and interfere at times with peak performance. Excluding the suicidal and the truly psychotic, these conditions are not dangerous.

Proper attention to bowel habits and prevention of mild heat exhaustion, simple as it sounds, will do much to make life pleasant for all. Rotation of tasks to relieve monotony is a great morale builder.

Extreme fatigue arising from long stretches of unruly weather, or the whirring of winches inches above your head during a long race that prevents sleep, raises the question of the use of sleeping pills. In my opinion it is contraindicated. When you get tired enough, you will sleep—in a wet bunk with the on-deck watch tramping overhead. And should you be needed for an all-hands maneuver, you will not be drugged and a danger to yourself and your shipmates. Leave the sleeping pills at home.

CHAPTER 9

Malaria

Con Tina, with the skipper and Betty aboard, returned to Cairns, North Queensland, Australia, after three months cruising to the Solomon Islands. Each person had taken malarial suppressive drugs (2 tablets of chloroquine) at 0900 every Monday morning while in the islands and for four weeks after leaving.

Five weeks after arrival in Cairns, the skipper, one afternoon, had a bunk-shaking chill, severe prostration, and a rapid rise in temperature to 104° F. Symptoms persisted only twenty-four hours. He visited the malaria unit of the Cairns General hospital where a blood smear was taken, but no malaria parasites were found.

Twenty-four hours later the skipper had another horrible chill and became very weak. A second blood smear was taken and again no malarial parasites were found. The laboratory explained that this often happened when the victim had been taking malarial-suppressive drugs.

Forty-eight hours later the skipper had a third chill. This time an extensive search of yet another blood smear found what looked like "malarial plasmodium." On this basis, with the skipper urging them, the doctors gave him adequate doses of quinine sulfate. He recovered.

This short case history illustrates the difficulties of malaria prevention and diagnosis, even when a modern hospital staffed by doctors familiar with the disease is available.

Malaria results from the bite of the female anopheline mosquito infected with one of the four malarial parasites: i.e., *Plasmodium malariae, vivax, ovale,* or *falciparum.* It was thought a number of years ago, following the discovery of the mode of transmission, that destroying the breeding places of the mosquito might conquer the disease. Unfortunately, this was not accomplished. Malaria is still one of the common causes of death in the world.

How did this happen? Populations got lax about destroying mosquito breeding places. The plasmodia developed new strains of parasites (particularly *Plasmodium falciparum*) that are resistant to suppressive drugs, i.e., chloroquine, so that travelers were suffering malaria attacks while taking these suppressive drugs. And the female anopheline mosquito changed her eating habits. She used to dine for one hour at dawn and dusk. Anyone who stayed behind screens for one hour at each time could avoid getting malaria. Not so nowadays—the lady anopheline bites any time the whim takes her.

New drugs were developed: Miloprim for prevention of malaria and Fansidar for prevention or treatment. These drugs were effective but sometimes proved toxic if given over long periods. Fansidar and quinine sulfate are both effective in treatment of malaria.

The best and safest method of preventing malaria is still under discussion by the experts. Medical research teams are working to discover effective, safe drugs. Other medical research groups are struggling to develop a vaccine similar to the smallpox and poliomyelitis vaccines to prevent malaria.

Fine for the future but, you ask, where does that leave me, a potential cruising sailor about to enter an area where malaria is endemic? Some knowledge of the nature of the disease is helpful. Malaria is practically two different diseases: one serious but rarely fatal, the other dangerous—sometimes fatal in a few days—particularly in the young.

The less serious malaria is caused by *Plasmodium malariae, ovale,* or *vivax.* The potentially lethal malaria is usually due to *Plasmodium falciparum.* This particular species of the malarial parasite family is most often resistant to chloroquine drugs taken for prevention.

We can only recommend the procedure we follow when traveling with grandchildren in endemic malaria areas. Many will disagree. If leaving from a U.S. port, contact the Centers for Disease Control (CDC) hotline in Atlanta. Before leaving a foreign port we try to find out as much as possible from local health agencies about what types of malaria are prevalent in the area we plan to visit and what treatment local physicians are using. Often the CDC suggests doxycycline as one of the drugs to use for prevention. Give it consideration. Aside from occasional photophobia it not only works well, but has few side effects and is not expensive.

What symptoms make the diagnosis?

Adult Malaria

1. Sudden, bunk-shaking, teeth-shattering chill.
2. Rapid rise of temperature to 103–104°F or higher.
3. Severe prostration, sweating.
4. Mental clouding.
5. Sudden subsidence of symptoms within twenty-four to forty-eight hours.
6. Recurrence of all symptoms in another twenty-four to forty-eight hours.

7. If the victim has had a previous attack he will make his own diagnosis with the first chill.

Child Malaria
The symptoms may resemble those of an adult or instead be only:

1. Fretful or disturbed behavior.
2. Fever of 102–104° F, often without a distinctive chill.
3. Marked weakness.
4. Convulsion if rapid rise of fever.
5. Abdominal pain and tenderness in left upper abdomen (enlargement of spleen).

Treatment of Malaria
The definitive treatment of malaria—both prophylactic and after onset—is under frequent change. It varies by region and type of disease. The best approach is to contact the CDC before a voyage to a malaria area and stock the appropriate medicine. Don't forget the prophylactic use of the drugs! If ever *prevention* is better than treatment, it is with malaria. This little piece of advice can save your life!

It is evident the diagnosis of malaria in a child can be difficult. Although it doesn't sound scientific, perhaps you might elect to follow the course of back-country hospitals in the Solomon Islands and Papua New Guinea (where 80 percent of children have malaria at some time in their growing up): A child under fifteen years of age admitted to a hospital with a temperature elevation above 101° F, regardless of symptoms, is immediately treated for malaria without waiting for blood smears. This usually works, as malaria is usually the cause of the illness. The bottom line is then in a so-called "malaria area," a sick patient with an undiagnosed fever must be considered to probably have the disease. Under these circumstances we have a clinical diagnosis of malaria and even without a laboratory diagnosis we should treat the patient for malaria.

A rough and ready medical technique you might wish to try (adults only) is that employed by many non-natives/Westerners who live for long periods in malaria-infested areas. They take no suppressive medication, but protect themselves from mosquito bites by various sprays, screens, etc. When they get an attack of malaria, they insist, and we agree, there is never any question in mind when it occurs, they treat it with quinine or the other drugs. Many of them say the suppressive drugs don't make you feel your best.

If you treat an adult or a child for malaria while cruising off soundings, keep a careful record of the kinds and amounts of drugs given. All such victims should be taken to a shoreside hospital at the first opportunity. The information as to the drugs given will enable the physician to give proper treatment to prevent recurrent malarial attacks.

It is evident that malaria is a serious and, in certain instances, a fatal disease. The foregoing presents a safe and plausible method of management if you are called upon to do this on your own. But evacuation to a hospital is desirable as soon as feasible.

CHAPTER 10

Miscarriage at Sea

4 June, 0700: Mike and Susie leave Rabaul, New Guinea, in their cutter, *Aubain,* round Gazelle Point, and head for Thursday Island in the Torres Straits. Distance—1,257 miles; E.T.A.—20 June.

6 June: Susie's expected menstrual period fails to arrive. She's usually prompt. This worries her a bit.

13 June: Susie suddenly has to visit the head every ten minutes. Her breasts are swollen and slightly tender. She's pretty sure she is pregnant. Mike is both pleased and worried when she tells him.

23 June: They arrive at Thursday Island. Pregnancy tests at the hospital confirm the diagnosis. There follow several days of decision making. Doctors are noncommittal as to whether or not they should continue their journey. Finally, Mike decides he could handle *Aubain* alone if necessary and they decide to continue their circumnavigation.

1 July, 0700: They head *Aubain* into the Torres Straits, to start for Cocos Island in the windy Indian Ocean. Distance—2,761 nautical miles; E.T.A.—27 July.

9 July, 0800: Susie's brushing her teeth—suddenly she vomits. She feels a bit better and stands her watch. There's a good reaching breeze and the steering vane is doing all the work.

———, 1600: She feels better: has skipped lunch, but takes a bit of nourishment now. Mike takes a fix—they have gone 1,044 miles, which leaves 1,717 yet to go to Cocos.

10 July, 0730: Susie wakens violently ill. After vomiting she still feels miserable, and Mike knows there are no medicines that would be safe to give a pregnant woman for nausea and vomiting.

11 July, 0003: Susie takes midwatch.

———, 0230: Susie can't stay awake in spite of coffee and taking off and putting on her clothes. A flying jibe rattles the rigging and tumbles Mike out of his bunk. They heave-to until daylight to check the rigging for damage.

11 July, 0600: Susie's still nauseated; Mike gives her some cola and some saltines. She drowses in the cockpit "on watch" while Mike hoists up and tightens the bolts on the starboard spreader tang. He comes down battered but intact and goes below to rest.

————, 1100: Mike takes over the watch. Susie, still drowsy but less nauseated, serves some coffee and biscuits and then folds up on her bunk. Mike stays in the cockpit dozing and waking until 2000, when the wind picks up a bit. Susie is dead asleep. They heave-to to avoid another flying jibe.

12 July, 0800: Mike takes a fix—250 miles in the past three days, leaving 1,467 still to go. Their poor progress is partly due to fluky winds but also to time lost heaving-to when both are too sleepy to sail.

13 July, 1600: Susie takes the watch while Mike organizes a meal.

————, 1700: The wind dies. They flop around in a ground swell. Susie vomits again.

————, 1800: Mike takes the watch till 2400 when he can no longer stay awake, and they heave-to. He remembers saying at Thursday Island that he could hand *Aubain* alone, but he hadn't counted on worrying about a sick wife at the same time.

14 July, 0900: Wind 18 knots, broad reaching, wind vane functions well. Susie feels better and takes some soup.

15 July, 1200: Mike gets a fix—348 nautical miles covered since the last position, 1,119 still to go to Cocos.

17 July, 1400: Susie goes off watch, and on her way down the ladder notices a bit of blood on her bikini—wonders if she isn't going to menstruate after all—a bit late. Then she recalls the nausea and pregnancy tests.

————, 1800: Susie develops more bleeding from the vagina and dull pain across her lower abdomen. Mike takes over the watch.

18 July, 0800: Susie has a sudden gush of bloody fluid from her vagina.

————, 2000: Susie's asleep. Then Mike gets very sleepy and decides to heave-to.

19 July, 0630: Susie awakes with severe cramps across her lower abdomen that radiate into her back. These come at regular intervals of five to ten minutes and last for a minute or so. She's having

steady vaginal bleeding, bright red blood. Mike is concerned, heaves-to, and gives Susie:

1. Demerol, 100 mg by intramuscular injection.

———, 1630: Susie's cramps increase, as does her bleeding. After one severe cramp, she passes a large blood clot with tissue. Bleeding continues, though somewhat abated. Mike examines the blood and tissue passed in an attempt to diagnose exactly what has occurred.

2. As it is reasonably certain, by gross examination of the material passed, that the tissue passed in addition to blood contained membranes and a fetus, Mike gives Susie 0.5 ml of Syntocinon by injection. He would repeat the Syntocinon 0.5 ml in ten minutes if bleeding had not markedly decreased.

———, 2000: "After-pain" and bleeding subside and Susie falls asleep.

20 July, 0800: Susie awakens hungry, thirsty, and with only a tiny show of vaginal bleeding. Mike feeds her and then gets a fix. Somehow, in spite of all the difficulties, they have made 150 nautical miles. That leaves a mere thousand, give or take a few miles.

1 August, 1000: They arrive at Cocos Island, clear immigration, and visit the doctor. He expresses regret at the lost life, but after pelvic examination, pronounces Susie in the best of health.

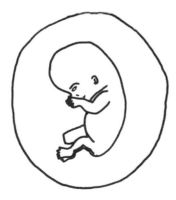

Fig. 38. Eight weeks' fetus. Actual material passed may be considerably distorted.

Later, over a beer, they make a solemn resolve. Birth control pills hold a higher priority in their traveling economy than beer or, perhaps, food.

10 August, 0800: They point *Aubain* westward towards the Seychelles, 2,562 nautical miles across the Indian Ocean; E.T.A.—30 August.

Discussion

Pregnancy is a normal bodily state and usually will go along without serious event. But not always, as Mike and Susie learned.

Frequency of urination is merely an annoying nuisance on a small boat with a crew of two. Nausea is a common symptom of early pregnancy which usually occurs upon arising, hence the common term "morning sickness." But it may happen at any time. Usually mild, it can be severe enough to require intravenous fluids to maintain water and electrolyte balance.

The cause of nausea and vomiting is a matter of speculation but it commonly occurs during the first weeks of pregnancy. Surely, the motion of a small seagoing boat aggravates the condition as Susie found out when they flopped around in the large ground swell. There are no medicines that may help relieve nausea and/or vomiting of pregnancy that the Federal Drug Administration has ruled safe for pregnant women. That is, the rare possibility always exists of the drug causing fetal abnormalities. Therefore, the old remedies such as saltines, sipping on cola over cracked ice and eating whatever you can tolerate is the way to go. Then too, early in pregnancy, drowsiness without any medication often requires many long hours of deep sleep. Obviously pregnancy should be considered when planning the voyage.

Minimal vaginal bleeding early in pregnancy usually stops spontaneously. Should it persist and increase, particularly if accompanied by tenderness over the lower abdomen and cramps, spontaneous abortion (miscarriage is a lay term) is threatened. A gush of bloody fluid and an increase of cramps, particularly if they are periodic, usually means miscarriage is inevitable.

The seagoing treatment for miscarriage is to allow the uterus to empty itself completely, for this stops further bleeding. An incomplete miscarriage (i.e., one with retained fragments of the product of conception) may continue to bleed for some time and raises the danger of infection. In this case, emptying the uterus was successful and the bleeding stopped; and, with the termination of pregnancy, all the other symptoms were relieved.

The bleeding in miscarriage may be considerable and frightening, but it is rarely fatal. Should it continue for long periods, the best that can be done at sea is to replace fluid by mouth and/or by intravenous or subcutaneous methods (see chapter 4).

There are many popular ideas as to the cause of miscarriage. Best informed opinion holds it due to a defective embryo. There is no scientific evidence to indicate that Mike and Susie's situation (i.e., on a sea voyage) had anything to do with causing a miscarriage. It is a medical opinion that a good egg is hard to shake loose. Many thwarted men and women who have tried and failed to cause illegal abortions by blows to the abdomen and various drugs will attest to that fact.

Douching or other means of emptying the vagina are condemned. The recently pregnant uterus is dangerously susceptible to infection which can be fatal, so stay out of the vagina. Sexual relations should also be avoided for two to three weeks after spontaneous abortion, and for the same reason.

What are the chances of miscarriage? Statistics show that at least 10 percent of all pregnancies end in loss of the fetus—usually in the early weeks after conception. In actuality, these statistics are probably low because many early miscarriages are never seen by a physician. The woman merely believes that she has had a delayed and somewhat heavy menstrual period.

Before the tenth week of pregnancy, the fetus and its membranes may be expelled intact. Mike was interested—even though somewhat upset to look at it—because he wished to know if it had been completely expelled. However, his exam by the "naked eye" was a "guesstimate" at best—and of very limited help. If Susie has minimal bleeding over the next few days, feels nonpregnant, and aside from some expected fatigue experiences no further difficulty, all is well. It would be wise for her to consult a physician at the next port of call.

Finally, this discussion presents no argument for or against contraception by any particular means. In spite of the fact that babies have been conceived and delivered on boats, in hedgerows, in the Outback, and at almost any time and place one can imagine, it is better, if you are a deepwater voyager, to plan to have your child when, for at least nine to ten months, you can interrupt your journey at a place that furnishes good obstetrical care.

CHAPTER 11

Spontaneous Pneumothorax

The crew of the cruising ketch *Achate* had been close-reaching from Rabaul, New Britain, to Madang in Papua New Guinea. On the fourth day out they were at 148°30′ east longitude and 4° south latitude, traveling on a port tack close-hauled. It was time to come over to the starboard tack to head directly for Madang.

Skipper Terry, fifty-four, was at the helm. Lois, forty, was below resting, waiting her turn at watch. Ian, the teenage boy they had picked up in Rabaul, went forward to bring the Genoa about as Terry put the helm over.

Suddenly, Ian screamed in pain, clutched his right chest, and slumped to the deck. Terry put *Achate* on autopilot, called Lois to take over the helm, and ran forward. Ian was:

1. Writhing on the deck, moaning with pain, clutching his right chest.
2. Gasping for breath.
3. Pale and sweaty, his pulse weak and thready.
4. Moving his right chest very little on breathing—his left chest was heaving.

Terry put his ear against Ian's chest wall (direct auscultation); his breath sounds were very faint and soft. He put his ear against the left chest wall and heard harsh, noisy, breath sounds.

It took Terry a moment to put all these observations together but then he knew that Ian had suffered a spontaneous pneumothorax. He called to Lois to bring 100 mg of Demerol in a syringe and give this to Ian by intramuscular injection. In a few minutes Ian's pain and some of his anxiety were relieved. Terry helped him to his bunk below, assuring him that he wasn't going to die in the next few minutes, a thought which Ian had been considering very seriously.

"Take it easy—let the Demerol do its work," said Terry. "You just had a spontaneous pneumothorax. Ever had anything like this before?"

Ian was too busy trying to get his breath to talk—he shook his head, no.

134

"You were born with a thinned-out bleb on the surface of your right lung. It just burst and let air from the lungs into the pleural space and partly collapsed the lung. The pain was due to the lung tear."

Terry took another look; Ian relaxed, mumbled something unintelligible, and drifted off to sleep.

Lois was impressed. "Where did you learn all that?" she asked.

"Did my homework," said Terry loftily. "Spontaneous pneumothorax is caused by rupture of a congenital bleb on the lung surface. It happens most often in the right lung and usually in males between fifteen and thirty years old."

"What can you do about it?"

"Usually nothing but sedation and reassurance. Most often the lung rupture heals, the air is absorbed from the pleural sac, and breathing returns to normal in a few days. The pain of the lung tear doesn't last very long."

"Is it common?" asked Lois.

"Somewhere between common and rare."

"Does it always heal itself?"

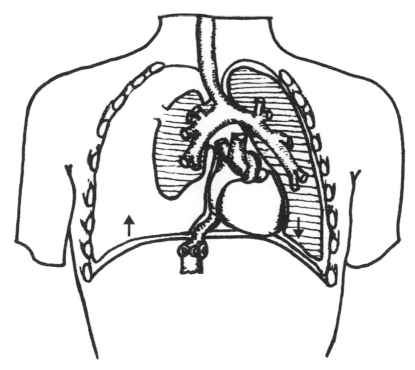

Fig. 39. Collapse of right lung after spontaneous pneumothorax.

"Never say always about matters medical," said Terry.

"What, then?"

"If the tear is too large to heal, breathing movements will keep pumping more and more air into the pleural cavity and increase the lung collapse. It'll also build up the pressure—a pressure pneumothorax, also called a tension pneumothorax. The air is trapped inside the chest."

"What then?" asked Lois.

"The pressure may press against the heart, great vessels, and the opposite uninvolved lung, enough to interfere with proper respiration and circulation."

"So?"

"We can't repair the tear in the lung, but we can let the trapped air out of the chest. Here's a description of the procedure, called thoracentesis, to do it. If Ian's breathing becomes worse and worse, instead of better, I won't want to do it, but I will."

Achate arrived in Madang three days later. Ian's breathing was gradually improving and in ten days he was feeling fine. He was advised by Terry to seek medical advice at the earliest opportunity because one attack sometimes means others might be coming along.

Technique of Thoracentesis

1. Sedate the patient with 100 mg Demerol intramuscularly if you have not done this in the past hour.
2. Put the patient in a seated position leaning forward slightly with his back facing you.
3. Draw 5 cc of 1% Xylocaine (see description of intramuscular technique in chapter 2) and with a small needle inject the skin muscle and underlying pleural sac with the local anesthetic (see # 4 below for injection site).
4. Insert the largest needle you have (a #18 is ideal) through the area of anesthesia into the chest cavity. This is done in the fourth or fifth interspace in the midaxillary line (a line drawn down from middle of armpit). Try to insert just over top edge of the rib, thus avoiding the major blood vessels and nerves which travel just under the bottom edges of a rib. You may feel a pop when you enter the pleural cavity. You can withdraw air in your syringe when you get to the right spot.
5. Suck out a syringeful of air.
6. Take the syringe off, leaving the needle in place covered with a pledget (pad) wet with antiseptic. Empty the air from the syringe.

7. Remove the pledget from the needle hub, re-attach the syringe, and draw off another syringeful of air. Continue this bailing as long as you can. It may take a while—there could be several hundred cc's of air. Don't be alarmed if a small amount of bloody serum accompanies the air. However, if you get solid blood, your needle is in a vein and should be moved a short distance backward or forward.

8. Withdraw the needle with a swift, straight motion and touch the pinprick with antiseptic solution.

9. Watch the patient carefully. You may have to repeat this procedure.

A patient who has had a spontaneous pneumothorax should be referred to a physician and a hospital at the earliest convenience. One attack indicates that others may follow.

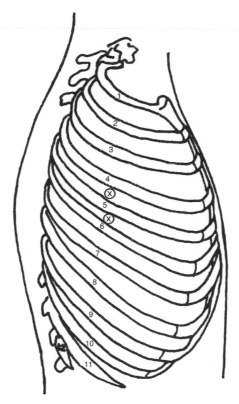

Fig. 40. Site of needle puncture for spontaneous pneumothorax.

CHAPTER 12

Inhaled Meat
(Café Coronary Disease)

Emma C, a 45-foot cruising ketch, had a rough interlude during the last three days of her ten-day cruise from Brisbane, Australia, to Port Villa in Vanu Atu. True to the prophecy in *Ocean Passages of the World,* viz., "It is rare to make this passage at any time of year without encountering at least one gale," a 50-knot wind hit them head-on three days from their destination.

Radio contact denied them shelter in New Caledonia or the Loyalties Islands unless they were in immediate danger. They were not. Wet, working hard, and tired they were, but in no actual danger. New Caledonia had been closed to visiting yachts for several months due to civil disturbances. Bill Junior had spoken with crews in Brisbane who had gone into Noumea without radio contact—they had been given a bad time by the authorities. *Emma C's* radio contact had warned them away. They decided to heed this warning.

The crew numbered four: Bill Junior, the skipper, and Sara, his wife, were both experienced cruising sailors in their late twenties; Bill Senior, Bill's father (age fifty), and Ian, a teenager picked up in Brisbane, were both on their first ocean cruise, and doing well. This fact helped Bill Junior decide to continue the cruise through the blow. Bill Senior had a special additional problem. A huge wave had caught him open-mouthed, head-on, and swiped his false teeth into the ocean. He had spares but they didn't fit comfortably. He planned to get a new set in Port Villa.

Cold and weary, they dropped anchor at Port Villa at 0200 on the eleventh day out from Brisbane. Crew and bedding were wet. This did not prevent immediate bunk time for all hands. They awoke about noon, dried their clothes, hung out the bedding, blew up the rubber dinghy, and put-putted ashore for dinner at Hotel Rossi.

The toasts flew thick and fast. Bill Senior drank martinis. Bill Junior and Ian downed a considerable number of beers. Sara preferred white wine. They drank to *Emma C* (sturdy boat), to Ian and Bill Senior (good performance on first ocean cruise), and then to each other and to the trip, and on and on it went. The crew was joyous to be in off the sea and anticipated a meal someone else would prepare and clean up after. They got a bit noisy but the other diners were tolerant, having seen a good many crews come off the big ocean.

Steak au poivre was ordered by all. When it arrived, the chatter was stopped instantly by the clatter of knives and forks. Bill Senior, chewing away, suddenly sat upright and grasped his chest, as pain twisted his face. His mouth worked furiously, silently. A dull, reddish blue colored his face—he slumped forward off his chair to land thrashing on the floor. Suddenly, he was still, except for twitching hands and feet.

"My God, he's had a heart attack," said Bill Junior, and headed for the telephone. "I'll call a doctor," he shouted back over his shoulder.

Sara had done her homework—she knew better. "Lift him up and seat him crosswise on the chair seat," she told Ian.

When he was held there, Sara stood behind him and clasped her hands together around his abdomen, just below the rib cage.

"Hold tight," she said to Ian. She put her knee into Bill Senior's back and gave a great heave with her encircling arms, pushing his abdomen up under his rib cage. Sara threw her whole weight into a second heave. Bill Senior's mouth few open and a glob of partly chewed steak flew out and landed ker-plop! in the bowl of soup of a man seated at the next table.

Bill Senior drew a long shuddering breath, his color returned, he coughed up a glob of mucus, and promptly vomited. Sara wiped his face with a napkin. He steadied on his chair and looked at her, gradually regaining composure.

"Holy cow," he said. "I was strangling and couldn't make a sound. You sure knew what to do, Sara. Thanks a million."

"You couldn't breathe or make a sound because you inhaled a hunk of steak instead of swallowing it."

"You can say that again. These damned teeth of mine. I'd better tend to my chewing from now on."

Sara didn't tell him that drinking may also have had a bit to do with his inability to direct air and solid objects to their close, but different, proper destinations in his throat, that this problem did occur regardless of teeth efficiency.

Bill Senior went off to the lavatory to finish getting himself cleaned up. The crowd that had gathered around began to disperse. Sara pushed her way to the soup goalie at the next table. He sat looking at the floating piece of gristle in his soup bowl—disgust wrinkled the corners of his mouth.

Sara explained that strangulation from inhaled chunks of meat, while not common, did occur, usually but not always in conjunction with drinking and faulty dentition. For many years, until autopsies became more common, this condition was diagnosed as a heart attack, hence the term "café coronary." A Dr. Heimlich had studied and devised the technique Sara had used: forcing the diaphragm hard up under the ribs to compress the lungs, which raises the pressure in the trachea above to pop the obstruction out.

"Sorry about your soup," she smiled. "Guess our aim wasn't too good."

"That's all right. It was worth it to learn about this condition," said the diner.

On a somewhat subdued note the crew finished dinner. Bill Senior's throat was a bit sore—he contented himself with some soup and a chocolate mousse. Bill Junior couldn't help repeated glances of love and admiration for his smart and wiry young wife.

The term "café coronary disease" is confusing. It is the condition of obstruction of the windpipe (trachea) and has nothing directly to do with the heart. It got this name tagged onto it because for many years it was believed to be a heart attack and naturally it occurred very often in restaurants.

The differential diagnosis (a fancy term which really means "What the devil is going on here?") between café coronary disease and a true heart attack is not difficult if you remember that the former sufferer appears to be choking but is silent. The material blocking his trachea (windpipe) allows no air past it to blow over his larynx (voice box) to make sound. Struggle as he may to breathe, he cannot make a sound or pass air in and out of his mouth.

The patient with a heart attack will groan, gasp, or yell with pain. Even though he, too, shortly loses consciousness and stops breathing there will be an interval when sounds and air can be observed or heard passing in and out of his mouth.

The treatment of café coronary disease is described by Sara's actions: Patient supported (most easily crosswise on a chair seat), operator standing behind, arms encircling the victim, hands clasped across the upper abdomen just below the rib cage, knee in the patient's low back, and a mighty heave to squeeze the diaphragm up against the lungs. This in turn raises the intrapulmonic (lung) pressure and pops the obstruction out of the windpipe like a champagne cork out of a bottle. It must be done quickly—death may ensue in a few minutes.

CHAPTER 13

Eye Injuries, Dental Emergencies, Otitis Media (Middle Ear Infection), External Otitis (Diver's Ear)

EYE INJURIES

Jeremy, forty-year-old skipper of *Wanderer,* a 40-foot motor sailing ketch, decided to take advantage of an unusually smooth passage from Avi-Avi to Malaita in the Eastern Solomons. The 15-knot breeze was abaft the beam, seas were slight, and the yacht slipped along quietly.

Jeremy fired up the generator, plugged in his power sander, and began work on the forward end of the port handrail which had been asking for treatment for some time. He didn't wear glasses (a serious mistake whenever sanding, grinding, or chipping).

After a few minutes' work he cut the power, laid down the sander, and came aft to the cockpit hollering to his wife Fran, who was doing the breakfast wash-up in the cabin below.

"Need help," he said. "Got something in my eye."

Fran wiped her hands, grumbling sotto voce about the number of times she had warned her husband about wearing safety glasses, and came up into the cockpit.

Jeremy sat on the edge of the cockpit cushion, his left eye scrunched up. He continued to rub it.

"Stop rubbing it," said Fran. "You'll make it worse; let me have a look."

She sat facing him, eyes at his eye level. The left eye was tight shut. Jeremy tried to pry it open without much success. Fran got a quick glimpse of reddened eyeball with tears spilling over the lower eyelid onto his cheek. After another try, she got a fair look by holding the lower eyelid out in spite of Jeremy's protesting growls.

She could see no foreign body. Must be up under the upper lid, she thought; that's a common location for dirt particles in the eye.

"Have to turn the lid," she said. Jeremy grimaced and shook his head.

"Don't worry, you big sissy," she continued. "I'll put some pontocaine in it and you won't feel a thing."

To care for Jeremy's eye, she:

1. Put two drops of pontocaine into the left eye.
2. Waited a few minutes until Jeremy's relief was evident.
3. Put a matchstick across the upper lid.
4. Grasped the eyelashes and upturned the upper lid.
5. Found a free-floating, sizable hunk of dark old paint in the middle area under the upturned lid, and deftly removed it with a moistened, twisted gauze wick.

"There," she said. "You'll be all right. But wear glasses until the numbness of your eyeball wears off or a seagull could fly right in and you'd never know it was happening. And if you go back to work, for heaven's sake wear the safety glasses. Next time you might not be so lucky."

"How come?"

"Hot, high-speed particles from chipping, sanding, or grinding can penetrate the cornea and become imbedded, and have to be removed with a sharp instrument called an eye spud, which we don't have and I couldn't use properly if we did."

"Suppose I'm stupid enough to leave off the glasses and get an imbedded one. What then?"

"You would have to wear an eye patch. We'd use ophthalmic antibiotic ointment a couple of times a day until we got you to a port."

"Would it be painful?"

"You should know. We could give you relief from time to time with pontocaine drops. But don't let it happen."

Jeremy nodded in agreement.

OTHER EYE INJURIES

The classic black eye or shiner is usually gained in personal contact with an opponent. This is not always the situation, though—the "I walked into an open door" variety does occur, too. These heal with application of a cold compress.

More severe blunt trauma may lead to hypemia (blood in the anterior chamber which appears as a bright red or dark fluid line between the cornea or outer covering of the front of eye) and the iris (the dark ring of muscle that furnishes those beautiful blue, gray, or brown eyes when uninjured). Treatment of hypemia is bed rest with the head elevated to encourage absorption of the clot.

Chemical injuries require thorough irrigation with eye wash, normal saline solution, or fresh water for five minutes.

A superficial scratch on the cornea may be painful but will usually heal if suitable antibiotic ophthalmic ointment is used to prevent infection.

Penetrating injuries of the eye with injury to and/or rupture of the globe and other structures are the most damaging to vision. In general, should such an injury occur at sea the best that can be done is to apply a comfortable dressing under an eye shield. Apply ophthomological antibiotic ointment if feasible and head for port or arrange evacuation. Control pain by oral or injected analgesics.

One-third of blindness in children is caused by trauma that is avoidable. Air rifles, arrows, darts, and missile-throwing toys can be left ashore.

Lacerations of the eyelid require exquisite plastic surgery to prevent complications of eyelid function. Application of a clean dressing will be better than any attempt to sew up such wounds. Head for port.

DENTAL EMERGENCIES

Two major dental problems arise at sea: severe tooth abscess spreading to the tissue of the jaw and neck, and a fracture of the jaw.

Dropped fillings and crowns are painful but not otherwise dangerous. A prepackaged dental kit, complete with instructions for use, will manage such situations. And, of course, proper dental prophylaxis prior to setting out on a journey will minimize lost fillings.

Broken teeth fall in the category of painful rather than dangerous injuries and pain medication plus a soft diet will prove sufficient.

A tooth abscess that extends may produce massive swelling of the cheek (if it be an upper tooth) or of the floor of the mouth and neck (if a lower tooth). The latter, particularly, may be a real threat, for soft tissues of the neck can swell to block the airway—a condition known as Ludwig's Angina.

Should a toothache and swollen lower or upper jaw develop:

1. Tap the teeth—the sore one will be the source of the abscess.
2. Give Cipro 500 mg three times a day for this serious and dangerous infection.
3. Give Tylenol #3 or Demerol 75–100 mg every four hours as needed to control pain.
4. Liquid diet.
5. Bunk rest.
6. Prepare salt solution (see chapter 4). Have patient hold this (as hot as possible) in his mouth against the sore tooth four times daily.
7. Discontinue medications when symptoms subside.

8. Saline mouth washes and antibiotics should be continued for a full week. If the dental abscess drains its pus spontaneously, or if all symptoms disappear, the patient will probably do well. If in doubt, continue treatment and call for help.

A broken upper jaw causes pain and disalignment of the teeth. Efforts to firmly close the teeth hurt, and it will be difficult for the victim to open his mouth wide. If there is obvious displacement of a segment of the jaw, a reasonable pressure to line up the teeth will do no harm.

1. Give a liquid diet as needed and Doxycycline 100 mg once a day for five days.
2. Administer Tylenol #3 or Demerol 75–100 mg by intramuscular injection every three hours as necessary for pain.
3. Stop medications and resume normal diet when pain subsides (two to three weeks).

Fracture of the lower jaw is complicated by difficulties of immobilization.

1. Give Demerol 75–100 mg by intramuscular injection.
2. Attempt to align teeth properly.
3. If there is bleeding from the gums at the fracture site (compound fracture), give Rocephin 2 grams by injection daily.
4. Fashion a jaw sling bandage to immobilize the lower jaw by fixation against the upper. Make it easy for the patient to remove in case he vomits.
5. If the patient can squeeze enough liquid diet through his bandaged jaw, have him do so. If this is too painful, pass a nasogastric tube (see chapter 6) and feed him a liquid diet with a bulb syringe.

Formula:
a. Powdered milk 4 cups after mixing with water
b. Eggs 4
c. Sugar 4 tbsp.
d. Vanilla flavoring

This provides roughly 1000 calories per feeding. Two or three daily feedings will sustain nutrition. Mashed potatoes, pureed soups—indeed, any food liquid enough to pass down the tube—may be added.

The patient may develop diarrhea. Give one Lomotil tablet with each feeding, but no more than eight Lomotil tablets in twenty-four hours.

6. Discontinue treatment when symptoms subside.

OTITIS MEDIA

Phil, the thirty-eight-year-old skipper of the 40-foot cruising ketch *Born Free,* together with his wife Annette and their two children, Robert and Ian, ages seven and four respectively, were one day out of Naifu in Tonga, heading for Suva. They were sailing comfortably along on a broad reach making between 6 and 7 knots in beautiful weather with a fair wind.

Robert awoke at dawn as he usually did when they were underway because he liked to watch the sun come up. This morning, however, he complained of an earache and was fussy, not his usual pleasant self. Annette examined him and found:

1. His face was somewhat flushed.
2. His temperature was 100°F.
3. His throat and tonsils were slightly reddened, not swollen.
4. The lobe of his left ear hurt when Annette pulled firmly on it.

Annette suspected trouble in Robbie's middle ear, but he had had earaches before which had not lasted very long or progressed particularly. He had not been swimming at Naifu because the water had been too cold. However, Annette was worried about the elevation of his temperature.

He continued to complain throughout the day and it was evident from his actions that the pain was getting much worse. In midafternoon Annette examined him. She found:

1. His oral temperature was 102°F.
2. His face was flushed with an anxious expression.
3. Gentle pulling on his left earlobe at this time caused severe pain.
4. When she asked him to chew a piece of bread, he did it reluctantly, stating in his grown-up baby language that this made his ear hurt worse.

She decided to give him Bactrim DS. Bactrim DS, one tablet two times a day, or Cipro 500 mg two times a day is a fine dose for an adult. Checking in chapter 18 she estimated a dose (lower) for this young sailor, and he was treated accordingly. In addition, she gave him a calculated dose of aspirin every four hours.

Towards the evening the good weather disappeared and a series of thunderstorms engulfed *Born Free.* There was considerable lightning and thunder and wind squalls chasing each other, one after the other, past the boat. Robert slept very poorly, complaining that the pain in his ear was becoming worse. At 0200, with Robbie fussing and his temperature now 103°F, Annette became very anxious knowing that without an otoscope she could not examine the ear internally.

"I'm glad now," she said to Phil, "that we took a subscription to MAS before we left the United States. There is nothing in the world I would rather do, at this point, than talk to one of their doctors who're on twenty-four-hour-a-day duty. It will relieve my mind to have some professional help."

"Fair enough," said Phil. He pointed to the horizon and the surrounding flashes of lightning followed by roars of thunder. "But it would be impossible for us to get in touch with MAS now—static would drown out any hope of radio transmission. We'll just have to do the best we can."

Annette comforted Robert as best she could, gave him another child-size dose of aspirin and made a hot-water bottle to put against the left side of his face and over his left ear.

After a restless night sailing through the storm with a child with a middle ear infection, Annette saw the weather clearing up next morning and made radio contact with a physician from MAS in the United States. He said that her diagnosis of middle ear infection was likely correct; her treatment of it was satisfactory and should be continued. He asked her to call back within twenty-four hours to let him know how the child was doing.

Annette continued the antibiotics, the aspirin, and the application of heat to the side of Robert's face. Toward afternoon he complained less and when she took his temperature it had dropped to 100° F. She made contact with MAS, reported this, and was told that she was doing the correct thing. She was also advised not to put anything in the child's ear. The doctor said the infection might progress to rupture the eardrum and allow a little pus to come out of the ear canal. If this happened she was to very carefully swab the outer end of the ear canal and not worry.

Robert's eardrum did not rupture. The pain subsided quickly—by the following day his temperature was normal, the flush was gone from his face, and the redness from his throat. A gentle tug on the earlobe was only slightly painful.

By the time they arrived in Suva, four days out of Naifu, Robert was his usual happy, childish self and apparently pain-free. They consulted a physician in the hospital at Suva who looked in Robert's ear with his otoscope. The drum had not ruptured. His left ear was in good shape.

Discussion

There are many causes for earache, most of which fortunately are not very serious. The commonest probably is a pressure phenomenon. The eustachian tube connects the oropharynx with the inner ear, inside the eardrum. This tube allows air pressure on both sides of the drum to be equalized. If it becomes obstructed the outer air pressure may be greater. This causes a stuffiness feeling, sometimes an earache. It is one of the reasons why, when a commercial plane is coming down to land, small children often cry—they don't know how to swallow to clear the eustachian tube. Modern airplanes, of course, are pressurized so this is not severe, but it does occur. Infection of the middle ear may be due to any one of a number of common infectious bacteria. It usually progresses via the eustachian tube into the inner ear structure. At first an infection causes swelling but it may actually go on to the formation of pus. Annette was very wise to start antibiotics early in Robert's illness because this did prevent pus forming, with subsequent rupture of the drum.

The land-based physician treating otitis media will of course have an otoscope to look at the drum and observe fluid accumulated behind the drum. Myringotomy (piercing the eardrum at the site of election in the inferior quadrant) may be done. If the child is in a situation where myringotomy cannot be performed, the drum may rupture spontaneously but not in the best location to prevent damage to the auditory ossicles (ear bones). This occurrence may or may not cause subsequent hearing problems. The damage will have to be assessed by a proper ear specialist at a later date.

EXTERNAL OTITIS

Earl, a thirty-seven-year-old skipper, and Barbara, his thirty-four-year-old wife, were taking advantage of a break in the weather to do some topside varnishing on their 46-foot motor sailing ketch, *Lanakoa,* tied to the remnants of the World War II military dock on the far end of Bora Bora.

Ginny, their ten-year-old daughter, helped for part of the first day then begged off to go skin-diving with her friend from a nearby yacht. She would disappear at or before breakfast, return only when darkness made further diving impossible, gulp her dinner, and tumble into her bunk.

One day Barbara noted Ginny was rubbing her right ear as though it itched. When she asked her about it she said it was nothing. Occupied with varnishing Barbara didn't pay much attention.

Several nights later, she heard Ginny, who usually slept like one dead, stirring restlessly in her bunk and moaning as though she were having a nightmare. Barbara woke her up. Ginny said her right ear was hurting. Barbara examined both ears:

1. The right ear canal was swollen, reddened, and had crusty discharge with some greenish pus. It was exquisitely tender.
2. The left ear canal was slightly reddened, but showed no swelling or discharge.

"You've had this for several days. Why didn't you tell us?" she asked Ginny.

"I was afraid you wouldn't let me go swimming," she muttered.

"Well, swimming is out for a while. You have external otitis media. Swimmer's ear, they call it."

"What's that?"

"Infection of the outer ear canal from swimming too much. Not enough time varnishing," she smiled.

"Can you fix it up?" asked Ginny, anxiously.

"Yes. But it's back to varnishing for you, young lady."

She then:

1. Squeezed a dollop of Neosporin antibiotic ointment and a small amount of 1% hydrocortisone cream into each external ear canal.
2. Plugged each ear with a cotton pledget.
3. Repeated this treatment daily for four to five days.

"If the cotton comes out of your right ear, come and let me put it back in."

"Okay."

"No swimming. And don't get your ears wet when you bathe or you may get into real trouble."

Ginny did as she was told. In addition, twice each day Barbara rinsed her right ear canal with dilute acetic acid to remove the crusts and discharge (vinegar 1 part, water 4 parts).

One week later, Barbara pronounced her cured. She allowed her to swim half an hour a day for a few days, then turned her loose. After each swim she had her rinse both ears immediately with a one-to-one mixture of rubbing alcohol and vinegar.

Discussion

This condition, which is popularly known in some regions as "Singapore ear," has plagued swimmers and divers forever. The normal outer ear canal is protected by a layer of wax. Extensive swimming or diving removes this coating and exposes the underlying skin and bone to bacteria. The skin is thin and stretched over bone and is vulnerable to infection. If neglected, infection may progress. The ear canal swells shut, and green pus forms. The skin around the ear swells; the lymph nodes at the angle of the jaw enlarge and become tender; fever indicates spread of infection, possibly into the bloodstream. When this occurs, systemic antibiotic treatment is needed. External otitis is often bilateral, so both ear canals should be examined. Barbara found no evidence of infection in Ginny's other ear but put the antibiotic ointment and cortisone into it just in case.

CHAPTER 14

Venomous Vermin of the Sea, Fish Poisoning (Ciguatera)

11 September, 0900: Pete is snorkeling along the reef at Cocos Island in the mid-Indian Ocean. Addie swims nearby. The dinghy they rowed from their sloop, *Wa* (anchored a mile away), is on the beach where they had shared a picnic lunch and a glass of white wine. Pete surfaces, feels a sharp stinging across his forehead, then, both arms and shoulders. He swims for the beach, some 50 yards away, alerted now, and dodging a second Portuguese man-of-war.

————, 0910: Pain clamps his chest muscles tight. He can't fill his lungs. He staggers from the surf, legs wobbling in an exaggerated goose step, and with a wild cry—"Help"—to Addie, collapses across the dory. He can't move his legs or get a breath.

Addie comes running. Quickly she:

1. Begins mouth-to-mouth resuscitation.
2. Pours the leftover white wine from their picnic over the welts on his back and shoulders (medicinal alcohol would have been better, but any alcohol would help).

————, 0920: Pete's breathing now, though he still can't move his legs. Addie rows the dory and its load back to the *Wa*. She stops twice on the way to resuscitate Pete.

————, 1015: Mike Thurston—whose cutter, *Destiny,* is anchored nearby—sees trouble and comes to help. Together, they hoist Pete's dead weight (he's still paralyzed) into the cockpit. Mike gets out the medical kit and gives Pete, by injection:

3. Adrenaline (1:1000) .5 cc,
4. Demerol 100 mg,
5. Phenergan 25 mg,
6. Decadron 8 mg.

He uses the same syringe and needle for four different injections—he does not mix the drugs. And, of course, he washes both

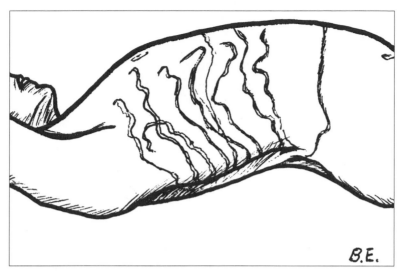

Fig. 41. Portuguese man-of-war stings.

the ampule and Pete's skin with alcohol before each injection. He would repeat the adrenaline .5 cc in five to ten minutes if Pete did not respond.

6. Addie slaps a thick paste made of baking soda and seawater on all the stings.

———, 1045: The paste dries and Addie scrapes the remaining tentacles off with a dull tableware knife.

———, 1055: Pete's breathing well, but deep muscle pain is only partly relieved by the drugs. The stings on his back now begin to burn and hurt.

Addie and Mike heat water in the galley—as hot as they can put their hands in—and dip towels and slap them steaming hot onto Pete. He objects, but they persist. Pain stops and Pete drifts off to sleep in a welter of soda paste and salt water.

12 September, 0800: Pete has only slight muscle stiffness in his chest and legs, and a back that looks as though he'd had a taste of the cat-o'-nine-tails (see figure 41). He's busily putting together an auxiliary first aid kit to take skin diving. It contains:

1. A resuscitating tube,
2. A pint of rubbing alcohol,
3. A dull knife,
4. A small package of baking soda,

5. Adrenaline (1:1000) (two 1-mg ampules),
6. Decadron 8 mg (two 4-mg ampules),
7. Demerol 100 mg (one ampule),
8. Phenergan 25 mg (one ampule),
9. A 10-cc plastic syringe and a sterile needle.

Discussion

The poison of the Portuguese man-of-war and of sea wasps is 75 percent as toxic as cobra venom. It is less often fatal because the delivery apparatus is less effective than cobra fangs. Nevertheless, extensive exposure is dangerous and can be fatal. The Portuguese man-of-war is not a single animal, but a whole seagoing colony of thousands of tiny cells clinging to a central floating stalk (see figure 42). Some members digest the food, some specialize in reproduction, but the dangerous ones are those with the long tentacles, the bases of which house the projectile nematocysts containing the poison. The venom can be discharged through the intact skin when the tentacle first attaches itself to the victim or later on, particularly if the nematocyst is stimulated.

This explains why Addie poured wine onto Pete's stings but made no immediate effort to remove clinging tentacles. Alcohol neutralizes the poison already discharged. A dilute vinegar solution or meat tenderizer can be used to destroy the venom. The baking soda-seawater paste should be left on to cover the sea nettle stings for ten minutes; then

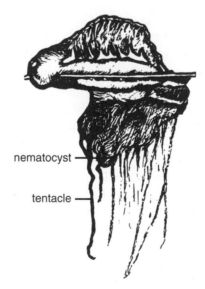

nematocyst

tentacle

Fig. 42. Portuguese man-of-war.

dull-knife scraping used to remove those as yet undischarged nemato-cysts. Rough removal, as with wet sand or a sharp knife, or rinsing these tentacles with fresh water, would stimulate the remaining nematocysts to discharge their toxins. In the event that baking soda is not available, alternating dry sand and seawater can substitute.

The toxin is a complex combination of chemicals: 5-hydroxytryp-tamine (5 Ht for short) is a potent, deep muscle pain-producing sub-stance. The exact mechanism of action is unknown. The best opinion at the moment is that pain is due to sensitization of the nerve receptors by the drug. This drug also causes much of the local itching and burning at the site of the lesion.

Tetraethylammonium hydroxide (tetramine for short), another com-ponent of the poison, has a curare-like action that causes muscle spasm and paralysis. There are, in addition, a number of low molecular weight protein poisons in the compound.

This combination of poisons produces muscle spasm, paralysis, the bronchial spasm that stops breathing, and shock and collapse, as well as the local skin welts.

Demerol is given to control the pain which, in an extensive en-venomization, is agonizing. Phenergan, an antihistamine, combats the bronchial spasm to aid in breathing and also reduces the severity of the skin welts. The Decadron is thought by many to aid in minimizing vas-cular collapse and shock. Cortisone cream rubbed into the skin welts also reduces the inflammation and hastens the healing of these lesions.

Finally, the compound venom is heat-labile—a temperature of 120° F will render it harmless. The hot towels at 120° F (which is about as hot as one can stand) do this. You will not burn the skin except on a child before puberty or on the aged.

It is beyond the scope of this book to consider all the dangerous creatures of the sea. Sharks, barracuda, and other fishes can produce serious or fatal wounds to swimmers. It is best to maintain a shark watch when swimming in strange waters, particularly between lati-tudes 25°N and 25°S, although attacks by these fish do occur in other areas.

Stingrays cause a painful wound that is slow to heal, and (rarely) systemic collapse. The injuries occur most commonly when a swimmer dashes into the surf and steps on a stingray buried in the shallows. "Go easy in on strange beaches" is a good motto.

Spiny urchins do not attack unless touched or stepped on. Be careful of strange-looking rocks when swimming or diving.

A final word of caution. There are, particularly in the coral reef ar-eas of the world, many fishes that are poisonous to eat. Captain Cook described them many years ago and James Bond brought them to literary fame when he was nearly fatally poisoned by the venom of a puffer fish. If you plan an extended cruise, particularly in southern waters, and expect to eat what you catch, it is best you learn what is good and what is bad, ichthyologically speaking.

CIGUATERA FISH POISONING

A fish encyclopedia, unfortunately, will likely not warn you about another type of fish poisoning not limited to one species. Ciguatera toxin may be carried by many ocean fish in the Caribbean and southern Pacific coral island waters. Although rarely fatal to a healthy adult, the symptoms are very distressing and, since the toxin is slowly eliminated from the human body, may last for weeks or months.

The symptoms were first described by Dutch navigators in the southern Pacific islands (1706) and again by Captain Cook (1776) who fed some fish entrails to pigs that died shortly thereafter.

The cause was unknown, however, until Dr. Y. Hokama and his group at the University of Hawaii Medical School and Adachi, Miyahara, and other Japanese research workers found that the toxin was

Fishes likely to be infected with ciguatera toxins:
Caribbean Islands: snapper
Florida: grouper, snapper, kingfish, amberjack, dolphin, barracuda
French Polynesia: grouper, snapper, wrasse, surgeon fish, shark
Hawaii: jack, amberjack, wrasse, goatfish, surgeon fish, snapper, grouper, parrot fish

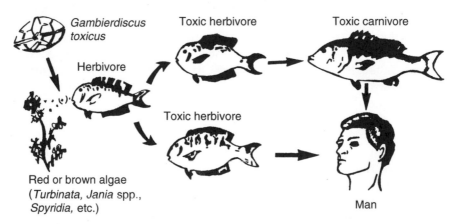

Fig. 43. Food chain for poisoning of humans with ciguatera toxin. Furnished by Dr. Hokama et al. from "Low Dalton Marine Toxins," *Laboratory Management,* April 1986.

carried by ocean algae (sometimes called the red tide). Figure 43 shows the food chain that infects people. Little fish eat the algae, are eaten in turn by larger fish, which are eaten in turn by humans, causing the infection.

The symptoms are of several types:

1. Gastrointestinal: nausea, vomiting, diarrhea (within 10 minutes to 24 hours), severe abdominal cramps.
2. Cardiovascular: rapid pulse with high blood pressure or slow pulse and low blood pressure (usually following in a day or two).
3. Neurological (nerve symptoms): headache, dizziness, numbness, hallucinations, temperature reversal, i.e., hot feels cold to the skin and cold feels hot (usually in five to seven days).
4. Neuromuscular: ataxia (difficulty in walking), loss of equilibrium (early, or in five to seven days).
5. Skin: severe itching, profuse sweating (early, or in five to seven days).

Symptoms may persist for many weeks, particularly the nerve symptoms. The poison attacks all ages and both sexes. The more fish eaten, especially gonads, roe, skin, and/or liver, the more severe the attack.

There is no known effective treatment. Immediate efforts should be made to empty the patient's intestinal tract. Vomiting may be induced. Treat with rest, fluids, and analgesics. Symptomatic relief of skin itching and perhaps helping the sufferer move to the head, etc., are all that can be done. Avoid alcoholic beverages, nuts, any fish or shellfish for two weeks following the poisoning. These could cause a relapse.

There are some suggestions (old wives' tales of doubtful validity) for ways to prevent poisoning. Small fish are assumed to contain less toxin, so may be eaten safely. (How small is small varies from island to island). On a more scientific note, there is also a new test kit advertised called Cigua-Check. Consult with your doctor about the latest available tests for this poison.

CHAPTER 15

Notes on Preparation for Cruising

You love your boat and never sail to far-off waters without a meticulous overhaul. But what about the people who man her? Spare parts may be easier to come by than spare crew where you are going. Your moral obligation to the safety and pleasure of the expedition demands maximum preparation of both. Each member of the crew should have a complete medical examination, and the results should be discussed privately with you.

A chronic disease need not exclude the sufferer but you must accept the added responsibility. For example, your potential port watch captain is diabetic. She has known and controlled it well for years and plans to provide her own medications and care. If you are willing to learn to manage diabetic coma and insulin shock, take her along. If you cannot, replace her. Another has hypertension (high blood pressure) but it is mild and uncomplicated. Do not worry about him except to remember he is not the best candidate for a stressful task. Duodenal ulcer disease may plague another. Present status and possible complications discussed with the man and his physician assure you that his routine medications and those necessary for an emergency are carried by that person himself and these precautions will prevent trouble. Crew members should carry ample supplies of any prescription drugs they use on a regular basis, as well as any drugs advised by their physicians for emergencies.

These few examples from a multitude of possibilities illustrate the principle of prevention by preparedness. But what about yourself, Skipper? You are the hub about which the whole wheel revolves—have your doctor poke and prod you until he is sure no unsuspected dry rot will collapse you. Ask him his thoughts about an elective appendectomy. If you or any of your crew have gallstones, surgery should be considered.

Emotional instability leads to problems on long cruises. Unfortunately this is often difficult to predetermine; most physicians are reluctant to expose their patients' neurotic traits. You will have to do a bit of discreet probing. A background of difficulty in dealing with proper authority, frequent alcoholic binges, numerous changes of occupation and/or wives might make you wonder if a certain fellow is just the man you want on watch as you dodge among the reefs and atolls of the Gilbert Islands.

Many sailors drink; some drink a lot. In my opinion, it is the question of *when* a person drinks—when the work is complete, or when he should be sober and on the job—that is important. Many times the choice is difficult. Balance personal charm and sailing expertise against immature irresponsibility of character.

Regrettably, drug and alcohol usage is too common. It is doubtful you will ever find a hard-core addict (heroin, Demerol, cocaine) seeking a berth for a long ocean race or cruise, but some sailors are frequent marijuana smokers and some use so-called recreational drugs.

Your only concerns are the safety and pleasure of your cruise. Avoid the popular argument, i.e., whether alcohol or marijuana is the "safer" drug. Poor timing in the use of any drug (including alcohol) may warp judgment when it should be keen. Continued excessive use of any drug (including alcohol) leads to serious defects in judgment and courage. The argument is practical, not moral. A wise skipper will not tolerate use of any drugs considered illicit unless they are prescribed for a specific reason by a competent physician. Alcohol use should be limited to "happy hour" or specific times decided upon by the skipper.

A balanced diet (protein, calories, minerals, and vitamins) is as essential to top crew performance as proper sail trim is to beating to weather. Vitamin C is particularly important since man neither makes nor stores it. Evidence strongly suggests that greatly increased amounts (up to 1000 mg a day) are needed for maximum emotional and physical performance under stress long before scurvy is apparent.

Certain other hazards threaten the unwary. The first week the non-manual laborer is at sea, his hands will be so sore from handling lines as to make them practically useless. Plan on this.

Don't go up the mast on a single halyard. Don't go swimming without posting a shark lookout. Don't cook with deep fat ever (fire hazard), and don't have boiling liquids on the galley stove while underway. The list of don'ts is endless, but ignoring the foregoing ones has led to many accidents.

One word about sanitation. People get smelly if unwashed and, more importantly, often suffer painful boils and other skin infections. Tap your heat exchanger or other engine cooling system for hot water, and wash with germicidal soap at least twice a week. Or, heat water on the galley stove to sponge-bathe. Brush your teeth to prevent cavity inspired toothache.

CHAPTER 16

Medical Prognosis—A Useful Art for Sailors

You are cruising Baja near Magdalena Bay in your trawler, *No Sudor,* with your wife, eighteen-year-old son, and sixteen-year-old daughter. A sudden lurch pours a kettle of boiling soup onto your wife's chest and abdomen, or perhaps tosses your daughter through an open hatch to break an ankle. Or possibly, on a sparkling Tuesday morning, son John skips morning chow—an unusual event—and complains of abdominal pain.

Unpleasant to think about, yes. Like storms at sea, accidents and illnesses, though rare, do occur. And just as good seamanship will get you through a major blow in the best possible shape, so some knowledge of what to expect from a particular illness or injury will bring you and your crew through in the best possible condition.

Medical prognosis is the art of predicting the future course of a given accident or illness. It's useful for the cruising or racing skipper. Although prognosis is difficult, if background information is applied with the courageous common sense usually displayed by deepwater sailors, it will help when trouble comes.

This chapter provides such information in everyday terms. It won't make you a doctor, but it may help you in the same way that an engineering manual will help you start your stalled Perkins 2,436 diesel engine far out at sea.

This discussion provides no treatment for any particular sickness or injury. Details of emergency medical care at sea are set down in many articles and in the preceding chapters of this book.

After you have done the fast first aid maneuvers, i.e., restored breathing, stopped major bleeding, and gotten the victim out of further danger, questions arise. Is this a serious injury? What is likely to be the eventual outcome? Do I need help or can I manage? If I need help but can't get it in a hurry, what can I do for the patient?

FRACTURES

Fractures may be simple (i.e., no wound in continuity with the fracture site) or compound (there is a wound in continuity with broken bone ends). Each presents different prognosis and treatment.

It is obvious first off that unless there is marked angulation of the part, you can't be sure there is a broken bone. However, if there is a severe sprain type of injury, it will do no harm to treat the injury as a fracture, provided you pay proper attention to the splinting.

Fracture of a finger, wrist, forearm, arm, lower leg, or ankle, when correctly aligned and splinted, can be cared for satisfactorily aboard for several days to a week. It is advisable to get help, but little harm will be done by an unavoidable delay of five or ten days. If there is to be a longer delay—two weeks or more—and if the shipboard reduction has been incomplete, a refracture may be needed later. This will prolong disability but does not exclude a satisfactory long-term result. Meanwhile shipboard splinting makes the victim comfortable and minimizes further injury to soft tissue from the broken bone ends.

Fractures about the elbow and extensive fractures at the ankle may interfere with the circulation of the arm or foot beyond the fracture site. Attention to general alignment and proper splinting are essential to avoid this.

A simple fracture of a long bone properly splinted, or a compound fracture washed up and splinted, requires many weeks to heal and although medical care is desirable as expeditiously as possible, unavoidable delay of a couple of weeks need cause no serious anxiety.

Fractures of the clavicle and of the ribs will heal without exception. If enough ribs are broken to cause a flail chest (that is, there is enough interference with the rigidity of the chest wall so that the lung will not expand when a breath is taken), this threatens life. Strap the patient's chest with wide adhesive tape strips all around.

Compound fractures (those with an open wound in continuity with the fracture site) present an entirely different problem. Unless the open wound is properly cleaned, it permits infection of the bone ends (osteomyelitis) and this will greatly hinder healing. If there is to be a delay of more than six to eight hours in evacuating a patient with a compound fracture, you can prevent osteomyelitis by wash-up of the wound and splinting of the extremity, plus systemic antibiotic therapy. There is greater urgency in evacuating such a patient than one with a simple fracture. The wound must be dressed frequently to keep it clean and sweet-smelling.

BURNS

Burns are deceptive injuries. A large second-degree burn involving a chest and abdomen with blisters and redness, but preserving sensation to pinprick, is a painful and terrible-looking injury. However, if it is less than 20 percent of the body's surface and infection is prevented, it can be treated successfully aboard and will heal. It need occasion little alteration of cruise plans.

Burns of second or third degree involving more than 20 percent of the body's surface as determined by the Rule of Nines (see figure 27; figure 54 for children) may develop burn shock eight to twenty-four hours after injury. If medical help can be gotten within that time, it should be. If not, heroic efforts must be made on board if the burn patient is to survive.

Third-degree burns of more than 10 percent of the body's surface, or an extremity, can be extremely serious, since such wounds result in a complete loss of skin and do not heal without a skin graft. Medical facilities are essential for this and evacuation within a period of days is desirable. However, if the wound is properly dressed, a delay of two or three weeks will not greatly increase the eventual disability.

Severe local third-degree burns, such as charring of an extremity (which is rare except with flame burns), often result in the dead tissue of the burned part forming a nidus (nest) for spreading infection. If evacuation is not possible, systemic antibiotics and meticulous dressing of the wound may reduce the danger.

Sunburn rarely causes dangerous symptoms except in redheaded persons with a minimum of skin pigment. Even when blisters develop, unless severe infection ensues, recovery with no aftereffects is the rule.

ABDOMINAL PAIN

Abdominal pain is a common complaint—usually not serious unless it persists. A surgical aphorism states that a previously healthy person who develops severe abdominal pain that lasts for more than eight hours probably has surgical abdominal disease. The rectal suppository is a useful diagnostic aid, since constipation—particularly in the young—is a common cause of stomachache. A rectal suppository does no harm and may resolve the problem.

The most common surgical disease of the abdomen is acute appendicitis, particularly, though not exclusively, in the young. Cholecystitis or gallbladder infection is a middle-distance second. It most often strikes the overweight middle-aged individual. Perforated duodenal ulcer is a distant third. There are many other causes for abdominal surgical disease, but statistics indicate that you are most likely to encounter one of these three.

A history of appendectomy eliminates appendicitis. It sounds obvious, but don't forget to ask first off! Persons with gallbladder disease usually have had prior trouble that may range from mild indigestion and intolerance to rich food to a severe colic with previous major abdominal attacks.

Perforation is unlikely to be the initial symptom of duodenal ulcer disease. A recent or remote history of treatment for ulcer by a physician will help make a diagnosis. A history of pain around the umbilicus when the stomach is empty (hunger pains) that is relieved by food or antacids points toward uncomplicated ulcer disease (see chapter 6).

The pain of abdominal surgical disease usually starts distributed over the abdomen and in the course of hours localizes over the affected organ which then becomes tender when pressed upon. Tenderness in the right lower abdomen points to the appendix; in the right upper abdomen at the edge of the rib cage, to the gallbladder. Pain of appendicitis is often gradual in onset. That of gallbladder disease may be gradual or severe depending upon whether or not a gallstone plugs the ductal system. If the latter happens, severe colic may start the attack. Perforation of a duodenal ulcer presents a dramatic event—sudden overwhelming pain around the umbilicus, often a shocklike state, and the rapid development (in minutes to hours) of generalized tenderness and a rigidity of the entire abdomen called "board-like abdomen." The abdomen thumps exactly like a board.

You aren't likely to become a diagnostician from these few observations. However, you can decide with reasonable assurance whether you are dealing with a medical abdominal disease such as dysentery, "intestinal flu," dietary indiscretion, or a surgical condition. Fortunately, shipboard treatment for surgical abdominal disease (detailed elsewhere) is similar regardless of the cause. It also is essentially harmless should your diagnosis be incorrect. So, it is wiser to overtreat rather than undertreat.

A word of warning. Attempt no abdominal operation at sea. You may have read of heroic "appendectomies" performed by laymen or paramedics on ships at sea. These are all near-disasters. The victims may survive in spite of, and not with the aid of, such ill-advised attempts. Surgical abdominal disease need not be fatal if an immediate operation is not performed. If the body's defense mechanisms are supported, as you can do, the patient can arrive in port in salvageable condition.

HEAT EXHAUSTION AND HEATSTROKE

Heat exhaustion is an acute condition due to excessive loss of salt and water from the body. Satisfactory replacement is possible without interruption of the cruise.

Heatstroke is an acute, dangerous condition. Treatment must be begun immediately, prompt recovery is sought, and protection from heat and sunlight for the remainder of the voyage is necessary for the victim of heatstroke.

DISLOCATIONS AND SPRAINS

Finger and toe dislocations can be reduced readily, particularly shortly after injury. Shoulder dislocations require drugs and more complex maneuvers, but reduction is possible.

Ankle sprains, properly taped, will support light duty. Any dislocation or sprain may have an accompanying fracture. If this is small, that is, without gross angulation, it will not be diagnosed without an X-ray examination. It never does harm to treat a severe sprain (massive swelling, severe pain, and discoloration) as though a fracture were present. If recovery is complete within three to four weeks from a severe ankle sprain, it is unlikely that fracture was present.

WOUNDS

Soft-part wounds are of great variety. Those resulting from sharp instruments present clean cuts with regular margins. After hemostasis (stopping the bleeding), proper wash-up, and closure of the skin, evacuation is not urgent unless major tendons or nerves have been cut. Inability to raise the fingers suggests transection of the extensor tendons at the wrist or hand. Inability to bend the fingers suggests a division of the flexor tendons at the wrist or hand. Numbness of the palm, thumb, and first three fingers suggests a transection of the median nerve at the wrist.

Such nerve and tendon injuries are best repaired within two to three weeks of injury. Merely clean and close the wound over these structures. This gives the surgeon a healed wound to work through later on and is most desirable. As a matter of fact, many surgeons presently prefer to close the wound, allow it to heal, and do the repair of major nerve and tendon injuries after an interval of from two weeks to two months.

Jagged, irregular wounds of crush or tearing type, particularly if the skin is avulsed (torn off) should not be closed. After a good wash-up, pack them open. Evacuation of the patient is then desirable, because repeated dressings of such wounds is difficult and time-consuming. These patients also require systemic antibiotic treatment.

Any wound, clean, lacerated, or rough-jagged, may become infected. Evacuation becomes pressing in these cases since the problems of wound care and the possibility of systemic infection are present and require complicated treatment.

HEAD INJURY—THE UNCONSCIOUS PATIENT

Head injury accompanied by loss of consciousness is always of grave concern and a rough estimate of the extent of the brain damage is gained by the length of period of unconsciousness. After consciousness returns, complications may develop in the days following. Persistent and increasing headache, fainting or violent vomiting without nausea indicate force-10 weather ahead for the sufferer and urgent need for neurosurgical care.

Any crewman who is persistently unconscious from head injury, high fever, or whatever cause, cannot be well cared for aboard a small vessel. You must immediately supply fluids parenterally, keep the airway clear of mucus, and provide for urinary drainage and, often, fecal incontinence. It is a major task in a hospital with all facilities. In my opinion, this situation urgently requires evacuation of the patient.

HEART ATTACK AND PENETRATING CHEST WOUNDS

These catastrophes require major hospital facilities as soon as possible. Certain fundamentals of care are available if evacuation of the patient is impossible. The patient with either of these conditions should be treated as a bunk patient until he can be moved to a medical facility.

CARDIAC ARREST

If your efforts succeed in restoring heart action, the same rule applies as for patients with a heart attack.

SEVERE INFECTIONS

Serious bronchitis, pneumonia, and throat and urinary tract infections are characterized by general malaise, often chills and high fever, plus symptoms pointing to the organ system involved. Cough, chest pain, and shortness of breath indicate serious pulmonary disease—likely pneumonia. A red sore throat with pain on swallowing, often with enlarged lymph nodes in the neck, indicates severe sore throat. Similar general symptoms together with frequency, urgency, and burning on urination suggest bladder or kidney infection.

Such persistent illnesses with temperatures of from 102° F to 103° F by mouth for two days indicate an infection that merits trial of antibiotic therapy (see chapter 7) and may be successful before help arrives. Failure of response to antibiotics may indicate a viral infection that will not respond to antibiotic drugs.

SEXUALLY TRANSMITTED DISEASES (STD)

STD are prevalent in our culture. These can be treated by proper antibiotic therapy aboard, but a test for the AIDS antigen and a follow-up examination when reaching home are essential.

CHAPTER 17

First Aid Kit

Considering what equipment, instruments, and medications should be carried on a voyage of any duration is almost an impossible task. To be fully prepared one would need the space, supplies, and expertise of a tertiary care emergency room, backed up by all the facilities of a great teaching hospital. Being reasonable and practical, however, one should consider the following:

1. The vessel should be equipped with a good communication system. Be it VHF-UHF, cellular telephone, telephone communication through the INMARSAT satellite system, or whatever variations are on line, it is critical that you and your crew have a plan on how to use the vessel's equipment for emergencies. There must be more than a "911" mentality. One must know how and to whom to direct the call to rapidly obtain the pertinent medical information needed. One may contact physicians from home or arrange to obtain help if and when needed from one of a number of sources such as AEA Worldwide Emergency Assistance, Medical Advisory Assistance, or the Johns Hopkins Access Line (see the textbook *Wilderness Medicine* for additional information concerning emergency resources).
2. The skipper should always have an evacuation plan in mind—i.e., routes to be taken to obtain help in life-threatening emergencies and methods for contacting Search and Rescue, Coast Guard units, etc. in whatever part of the world he or she is traveling.
3. The skipper should be aware of any chronic medical problems that a crew member has. A frank discussion of these limitations with medication guidance should be had before this individual is accepted for the voyage. There are risks for all of us going to sea, but some bring problems with them that bear special consideration. What about the person on Coumadin (a blood-thinning agent) to prevent stroke because he or she has significant cardiovascular disease? Trauma to this person could be fatal. Equipment to monitor blood Coumadin levels in these

cases or blood glucose levels in diabetes is not usual on any small vessel. Nor is an electrocardiography machine, a cardiac defibrillator, etc.

All of these special problems must be considered in selecting a crew, and the crew must realize the limitations of the first aid kit. Medicine has made tremendous advances in recent years, but all of these advances cannot be available on small boats.

You cannot design a first aid kit that is likely to get all used up. If the medical supplies you must stock were all consumed, it would have been a catastrophic cruise, indeed.

The quantities of antibiotic drugs recommended here are based upon a crew of eight for a cruise of a year or more, presuming each person may require treatment of one severe infection. Overlap and substitution provide a wide margin of safety if an unusual number of infections arise. The penicillins have been avoided because many require hypodermic injection, many people are allergic to these drugs, and the broader spectrum antibiotics provide wider coverage. The broad-spectrum antibiotics are particularly helpful when the number of "meds" must be limited.

Decadron, atropine, and Valium are among others you will carry and probably never use. Yet if you do need these they may be lifesaving.

Purchase your drugs and supplies at home before setting out. Be sure to get the longest shelf life possible on all medications. Consult your physician; he or she will need to furnish prescriptions which you must have for many items and, together with your druggist, may suggest alternate drugs or better methods of packaging than are available at the time of this writing. Generic drugs may markedly reduce your cost. Most "pills" come in large bottles, but you can get less than a full bottle. Sometimes there is a price break if you purchase 100 or more pills. Always insist on getting a package insert, that is, the manufacturer's information on the drug. The information could be lifesaving. Finally, note that familiar drugs travel under strange names in foreign countries. You might not know what to ask for if you wait until then to purchase them.

The urethral catheterization kit (see figure 33) and the dental kit are sterile, sturdily packed, and easy to stow. The plastic covers resist moisture so long as the seals are intact. Do not sterilize these for reuse by heat; it melts the plastic. Scrub the instruments well with Betadine and fresh water, then rinse and soak for two hours in an antiseptic such as rubbing alcohol.

Disposable syringes and needles (see figure 36) and soap scrub pads (see figure 44) are sterile and prepackaged in water-resistant, but not waterproof, paper. A glass or metal syringe with metal-hubbed needles should be taken too, because it can be resterilized forever.

If at all possible you should make room for liter bottles of prepared parenteral salt solution. You can make your own if you do not or if a sudden emergency uses your supply (see page 171).

We find plastic tackle boxes handy for drug stowage (see figure 45). There are many sizes, the shelves with convenient dividers fold out, and the boxes do not corrode.

DRUG LIST

The following list of drugs and supplies relates only to diagnosis and treatment of the serious emergencies discussed in this book. You will want a standard first aid manual and supply kit for the lesser problems.

For each item on the list the following information is given: the name of the drug and its action, how it is to be used, how it is supplied, and the suggested quantity to take on your trip. All drugs and supplies marked with an asterisk will probably require a physician's prescription.

When outfitting your kit, consult your family physician with this drug list in hand. You will need prescriptions. Be sure to tell the physician that you will use the drugs only when away from medical care and only on your own crew people. The physician can instruct you in the proper use of these drugs and supplies.

Prescription drugs are all packed with detailed information on usage, dose, and dangers. Please consult that information! The following

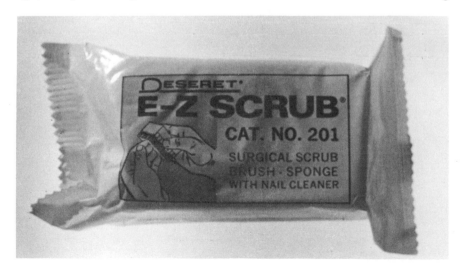

Fig. 44. Soap scrub pad.

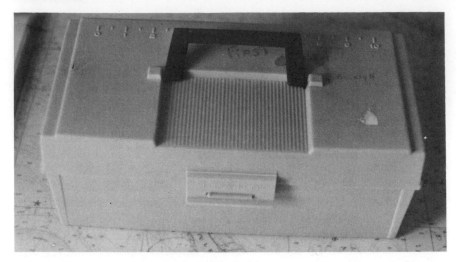

Fig. 45. Plastic tackle box first aid kit.

list is intended only to give some very basic information. Doses of drugs mentioned below are for the average 150-pound person. See chapter 18 for help in choosing the proper dose for a child.

A & D Ointment. For application to clear chronic sores and promote healing. Supplied as 4 gm tubes. Stock 2 tubes.

*Adrenaline HCL (1:1000 dilution). Potent adrenal hormone to inhibit severe antigen-antibody reactions such as anaphylactic shock or severe drug or allergic reactions. Consult package insert for dosage. Supplied in 1 cc ampules for injection. Stock 8 ampules.

Aspirin, 300 mg tablets. Stock 300 tablets.

*Atropine sulfate. A parasympatholytic drug that relaxes the gastrointestinal tract and the gallbladder. Supplied in 1 cc ampules of 1/150 gram for injection. Stock 4 ampules.

*Bactrim DS. A synthetic antibacterial medicine that is very useful for urinary tract and gastrointestinal infection. Supplied in bottles of 100; usual dose is 1 tablet twice daily. Stock 2 bottles.

Benadryl 25 mg capsules. Antihistamine with sedative actions. Supplied in bottles of 100; usual dose is 1 or 2 capsules every four hours for acute allergy or for insomnia. Stock 2 bottles.

Betadine skin cleaner. A topical antiseptic bactericide that may be used to cleanse all wounds and for washing the medical attendant's hands before handling open wounds. Supplied in 4 oz plastic bottles. Stock 3 bottles.

* Requires prescription.

Cavit. A packing for tooth cavity from a broken filling. Remove debris from the area by saline mouthwash, dry with cotton, and apply cavit. Obtain a small amount from your dentist or a dental supply house.

*Chloroquine. A malarial suppressive drug that may be suggested by the Centers for Disease Control for prevention and/or treatment of the disease in malarial areas. The type and amount of these drugs for malaria should be decided upon based on this advice before putting to sea.

*Cipro 500 mg tablets. A potent antibiotic with a broad spectrum of use; usual dose is 1 tablet twice daily. Stock 300 tablets.

*Claritin 10 mg tablets. Antihistamine. Usual dose is 1 daily. Stock 1 bottle of 50 tablets.

Cortisone cream 1% (hydrocortisone cream). Inhibits inflammatory reaction; excellent for contact dermatitis and various skin irritations. Supplied in 45 oz tubes. Stock 3 tubes.

*Cortisporin ophthalmic ointment. Contains two antibiotics plus cortisone and can be used for most eye inflammations. Please check the package insert. Oral antibiotics may also be used at the same time. Supplied in 3.5 gram tubes. Stock 3 tubes.

Cough drops. A wide variety of these are sold without prescription. Packs of several types should be stocked as they are often excellent for symptomatic relief.

*Decadron. Potent adrenal cortical extract used to treat poisoning, severe antigen-antibody reactions, and shock. Please refer to package insert before using to get correct dose. Supplied in box of 25 1 ml vials for injection and in .5 mg tablets. Stock one box of vials and one bottle of 100 tablets.

*Demerol. A narcotic for pain relief. Dose varies from 50 to 150 mg every four hours. See package insert. Demerol may be given with Phenergan by injection to enhance the drug's effects. Supplied in ampules containing 1 cc (50 mg) in sterile cartridge for injection. Stock 10 ampules and one 30 cc bottle containing 50 mg per cc.

*Doxycycline 100 mg capsules. An antibiotic for infections. Usual dose is one capsule every 12 hours. Stock one bottle of 100 capsules.

Dulcolax rectal suppositories. A safe and effective agent for constipation. See directions on box. Supplied 12 in a box. Stock 2 boxes.

Gelusil tablets. An antacid for indigestion. Supplied in various sized boxes. See package instructions for dosage. Stock 100 tablets.

* Requires prescription.

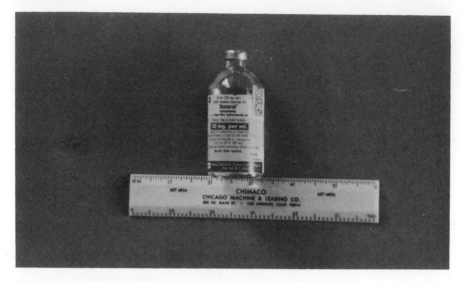

Fig. 46. Demerol in multiple-dose 30 cc vial, 50 mg/cc.

Ipecac. Potent emetic used to induce vomiting after ingesting certain
dangerous chemicals. See package insert. Stock 1 oz.

*Keflex 500 mg tablets or capsules. Oral antibiotic to treat infections.
Usual dose is 500 mg every six hours. Stock 300 tablets.

*Lasix. An injectable diuretic useful in heart disease as well as near
drowning in fresh water. Supplied in 100 mg ampules and 20 mg
tablets. Stock 3 ampules of injectable Lasix and 25 tablets.

*Lomotil tablets. Helpful to control diarrhea. Please read package insert
for information on when this drug should be used. Do not exceed 8
tablets per day for an adult and fewer for a child. Stock bottle of 150.

*Metronidazole 250 mg tablets. A potent antibiotic frequently needed
for gastrointestinal disorders. Usual dose is 1 tablet every 8 hours.
Stock 100 tablets.

Neosporin antibiotic ointment. This combination of polymyxin B sulfate, bacitracin zinc, and neomycin sulfate is a very useful product
for skin wounds. Supplied in ½ oz tubes. Stock 6.

Oil of cloves. A counter-irritant. Place a few drops on a small piece of
cloth and insert in a painful tooth cavity. Stock one ⅓ oz bottle.

Pedialyte dry. Flavored powders containing electrolytes for treatment
of dehydration and electrolyte imbalance. Follow directions on mixing and use only by mouth. Stock 10 packets if children are aboard.

Pepto-Bismol tablets. An antacid for indigestion. Take as package di-
rects. Supplied in boxes of 30 tablets. Stock 3 boxes.

* Requires prescription.

*Phenergan rectal suppositories 25 mg. Excellent drug for motion sickness; can be used every eight hours. Supplied 12 in a box. Stock 3 boxes.

*Phenergan injectable. An antihistamine and sedative action make this a good adjunct to Demerol to treat pain. It may reduce the need for a narcotic dose by up to 50 percent. See package insert for doses. This can also be used in lieu of rectal suppositories for seasickness. Supplied as 25 mg/ml in 1 ml ampules, packaged in 25s. Stock 1 package.

*Pontocaine anesthetic eye drops. 1% topical anesthesia for the cornea and conjunctiva used for injury producing pain such as when a foreign body is in the eye. It is also used for excess ultraviolet radiation producing "snow blindness." Read the package insert. Stock .5 oz bottle.

*Rocephin for injection. A broad-spectrum antibiotic that can be given by intramuscular or intravenous injection whenever the oral route is contraindicated. See package insert for dosage. Supplied in 1 gm vials in boxes of 10. Stock 2 boxes.

*Silvadene salve 1%. Important topical treatment for second and third degree burns. Supplied in 400 gm jars. Stock 4 jars.

Sodium chloride enteric coated tablets. These coated salt tablets do not dissolve until they arrive in the intestines, hence preventing nausea. In tropical cruising where "sweating" is profuse, these help rebuild one's salt loss. See package insert for doses. Supplied in bottles of 100 tablets. Stock 2 bottles.

Sodium chloride, non—enteric coated. Regular salt tablets to make up into salt solution for parenteral administration after severe burns, shock, peritonitis. The number of tablets needed to make a quart will be on the label of the bottle. Take enough tablets to make four quarts of saline solution. If tablets run out, use 1 scant teaspoonful of table salt to one quart of water. If you have storage space, take 6 quarts of prepared, sterilized salt solution together with tubing, needles, and instructions for use. This may be given subcutaneously or intravenously. Do not add antibiotics to the salt solution given subcutaneously; antibiotics must be given by separate deep intramuscular injection.

*Syntocinon 0.5 ml for injection. An oxytoxic drug used to contract the uterus and decrease bleeding after miscarriage or birth. Supplied in ampules. Stock 6.

*Tagamet 400 mg. A drug that inhibits gastric acid secretion that is very useful in duodenal ulcer disease or heartburn that are resistant to antacids. Stock 40 tablets.

* Requires prescription.

*Tetanus toxoid absorbed. Necessary for use in puncture wounds, severe injuries, and burn cases to prevent tetanus. Supplied in 5 ml vials. See package insert for doses. Keep refrigerated. Stock 1 vial.

*Tylenol #3 (containing ½ gr of codeine) tablets. This oral narcotic is excellent for mild to moderate pain. Usual dose is 1 tablet every three hours as needed for pain. Stock 100 tablets.

Tylenol Extra-Strength. Strong analgesic for use when Tylenol #3 is not needed. Stock 2 bottles of 100.

*Valium (diazepam). Potent tranquilizer useful for controlling severe acute irrational behavior or convulsions. Supplied in 2 ml disposable syringes (each containing 5 mg of diazepam/ml), 10 per box. Stock 1 box. Also supplied as 5 mg tablets that may be used for children (adjust doses) or adults. Cut tablets in half as needed for child's dose. See package insert.

Vaseline. Petroleum jelly used to lubricate nasogastric tube or catheter before use or gauze for nasal pack. Stock 1 large jar.

*Xylocaine 1% without epinephrine. A topical local anesthetic. Supplied in 50 cc vials. Stock 4.

SUPPLIES

Ace bandage. Elastic bandage for pressure dressing on wounds, sprains, splints. Comes in 2", 3", 4". Stock 2 of each.

ADAPTIC (Johnson & Johnson) nonadhesive wound dressings. Stock 1 box of 12 dressings that are 3" × 3".

Alcohol sponges. Stock 1 box.

Baking soda. Stock 1 large box.

Bandages. Sterile gauze 1", 2", 3". Stock 6 of each.

BAND-AID brand (or other) adhesive bandages. Assorted sizes of bandages for simple wounds. Stock 3 boxes of assorted sizes.

Bulb syringe. Glass syringe of 2–3 ounces capacity with rubber suction bulblike douche syringe or turkey baster. Stock 2.

Cast liner. Padding for splints. Also useful for head and jaw bandages. Supplied in 3" rolls. Stock 4 rolls.

Catheter. Rubber tube with fluted tip to pass through urethra to empty urinary bladder. A Foley catheter has a retaining balloon. Prepackaged sterile, size No. 14. Stock 3. [There will be another (Robinson) in catheter kit.]

For a child, use size No. 8. Stock 1.

Compound tincture of benzoin. Adhesive liquid for external use before applying adhesive tape bandages. Stock 2 oz bottle.

*Requires prescription.

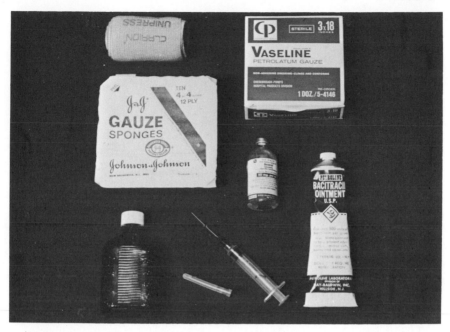

Fig. 47. Burn dressing kit.

Cotton absorbent. Sterile cotton. Stock 2 packs.

Cystotomy needle. 4" spinal puncture needle No. 18. Packaged in plastic container. Stock 2.

DRL 5% 1000 cc for intravenous or subcutaneous injection. Stock 8 1000 cc plastic containers of DRL 5%.

Forceps. Toothed and plain tweezers for various uses. Stock 1 of each.

Gauze. 4" × 4" squares—sterile, prepackaged in boxes of 10 (12-ply). Stock 8 boxes.

Graduated cylinder. Plastic cylinder, measured in ounces and cubic centimeters. Stock 1.

Hemostat. Artery-occluding forceps. Stock 6.

Hypodermic syringes. Plastic, disposable, prepackaged, sterile.

    Size 1 cc, insulin-type, with no. 25, ½" needle. Stock 6.

    Size 5 cc with no. 22, 1½" needle. Stock 24.

    Size 10 cc with no. 22, 1½" needle. Stock 6.

    Size 20 cc with no. 20, 3" needle. Stock 4.

    Size 50 cc with no. 18, 3" needle. Stock 2.

*Requires prescription.

Isopropanol. A 70% solution of ethyl alcohol used to clean areas near wounds, prepare areas for surgery, and as a rinse for the "surgeon" after washing up for a procedure. Stock one 16 oz plastic bottle.

KLING (Johnson & Johnson). An excellent sterile bandage to place over the primary bandage to hold the dressings in place. Supplied in boxes containing 5 bandages 3" × 3.6 yards. Stock 1 box.

Knife. Bard-Parker handle No. 3. Stock 3.

Knife blades. Sterile, packaged in plastic, No. 10. Stock 6.

Needle holder. Metal forceps with lock handle for holding a curved needle. Stock 1.

Resuscitating tube. Plastic airway for mouth-to-mouth resuscitation. Supplied in plastic bag with indelible instructions. Stock 1.

Soap pads. Scrub pads, sterile, prepackaged, individual. Impregnated with antiseptic soap. Stock 6.

Splints. Devices for immobilizing broken bones or crushed extremities. Cardboard; stow flat and fold up for use. Stock 3 adult.

Staple remover (WECK). Supplied 6 in a box. Stock 1 box.

Steri-strips. Adhesive strips for wound closure instead of sutures. Supplied as 6 strips per sterile, plastic package. Size ½ × 4". Stock 6 packages.

Stethoscope. An instrument used to listen to the heart, lungs, and to take the blood pressure.

Stomach tube. Plastic or rubber tube to pass through the nose into the stomach. Need not be sterile. Should be marked on outer end to indicate location of tip in stomach. Stock 2.

Sphygmomanometer (blood pressure cuff). An instrument used to measure arterial blood pressure, which can also be used as a tourniquet.

Surgical gloves. Disposable surgical gloves come in sterile packages by the pair in small, medium, or large. Stock 18 pairs.

Sutures (sewing thread). Packed in individual sterile envelopes. Attached onto cutting needle. Size 2-1 silk for tough skin can be used on most parts of the body apart from the face, hands, and any areas where the skin appears thin or delicate. Size 4-0 silk is finer and should be used for thin skin. Size 2-0 catgut (absorbable) is used in deep tissues. Stock 20 of each kind.

Thermometer (clinical). To record oral or rectal temperature. Sterilized by wiping off with alcohol. Stock 3 in metal cases.

Universal arm splint. Plastic splint for either forearm and wrist. Stock 1 adult size.

Vaseline gauze. Fine mesh gauze impregnated with Vaseline. Good dressing for burns, compound fractures. Does not stick to wound. Also can make sucking chest wound airtight. Supplied as boxes of 12 sterile, individual packs. Size 3" × 36". Stock 2 boxes.

Visistat stapler (WECK). Supplied as 35 staples with applicator device, 6 packs in a box. Stock 1 box.

As stated previously, the drugs and supplies described on the foregoing pages in this chapter are designed to equip a vessel with a crew of eight for a voyage of up to a year. For every boater lucky enough to enjoy such a cruise, there are thousands who must limit themselves to weekends or vacation cruises of a few weeks. Such cruises are usually planned within reasonable distance of supervised medical aid.

It cannot be sufficiently stressed that it is virtually impossible to plan for all the medical supplies one might need on a cruise. Generous amounts of supplies are called for in this extensive list, but something will always be lacking. In previous editions of this book abridged lists of medicines and supplies were given for shorter cruises. This editor saw a tragedy in the Arctic Ocean where one-third of the passengers on a cruise ship were casualties within a matter of minutes and all the medical supplies were exhausted within twenty-four hours. Conversely, there was a cruise to the most distant areas of the Antarctic with over a hundred passengers for many weeks and I hardly dispensed a pill. Therefore it seems inappropriate to use abridged lists. Should you feel that for expense and space limitations there is a need to cut back on the medicines and supplies recommended, discuss your specific needs with your physician and pharmacist.

Each crew member must carry medical supplies of the type they routinely use. Stressing this to your crew members is extremely important.

Lastly, this is a book for advanced first aid afloat. It makes no attempt to be a medical textbook. *The Merck Manual,* 17th edition,

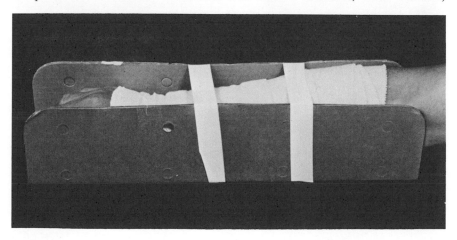

Fig. 48. Cardboard arm splint stows flat.

published in 1999 by Merck Research Laboratories, is an excellent resource. Its almost 3,000 pages come in a very compact, well-organized volume. Much of this book would be understood by you and some of your crew and might give you the background and reassurance necessary on an extended cruise. Putting the *The Merck Manual* together with this book onboard gives you a good compact medical library.

Again, it is advisable to go over the drug list with your own physician, since many of the drugs will require a prescription. He or she can show you proper technique for drug injection and, with a knowledge of your particular expedition, further help to determine the drugs and supplies you'll most likely need.

Care of the Sick or Injured Child

GENERAL MANAGEMENT, DRUGS AND DOSAGE

A child's different response to stress and lack of ability to give a coherent history, coupled with unreliable findings on physical examination (children are often inaccurate about what hurts and where), make first aid management of children difficult. There may be resistance to bad-tasting medicines and certainly to injections (this last not confined solely to children).

A child's body fluid content (60 percent of body weight) is similar to an adult's, but the child's smaller size means there is less total amount. Small losses from vomiting, diarrhea, or hemorrhage may rapidly lower circulating volume to critical levels. Replacement is urgent. Children require 25 percent of total fluid for replacement of daily losses (perspiration, vaporization in lungs, urine); the adult needs only 9 percent of total for this purpose.

Children suffer some serious diseases and accidents that adults encounter rarely or never. Bacterial meningitis, otitis media (middle ear infection), choking from swallowed or inhaled foreign bodies, accidental ingestion of poisons (many of which are compounds commonly used for boat maintenance), and drowning are examples that will be discussed in the following chapters.

Children are given the same drugs as adults with an adjustment of dosage based on age and weight. You must know your child's weight to make intelligent decisions about safe, effective drug doses and fluid quantities to give for advanced first aid management. You can lug along a steel beam scale but it demands too much storage space. A spring bathroom scale requires less stowage, but won't give you a much more accurate weight than the two methods we are about to describe, which require no extra equipment.

DETERMINING A CHILD'S WEIGHT

Method 1
When having your child's immunization schedule brought up to date prior to departure, have the nurse or doctor record his or her weight.

Consult figure 49 or 50 and find which of the seven curves fits your child's weight/age most closely. Mark it point A. Nine months later, as you approach the Solomon Islands, you can follow along the curve to arrive easily at his or her probable current weight.

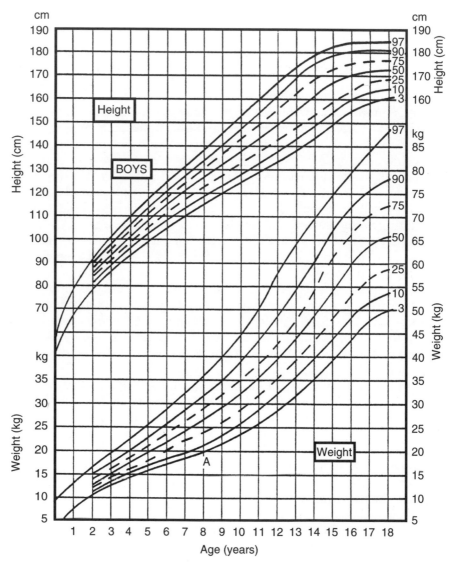

Fig. 49. Boys' age/weight curves. Courtesy Red Cliff Hospital, Red Cliff, Queensland, Australia, Dr. C. Pollard, Chief of Surgery.

Example

Johnnie is eight years old; he fits on the lowest age/weight curve (20 kilograms). Not to worry—all seven curves are for normal children allowing for build, etc. Nine months later you find, using figure 49, that he has gained 1 kilogram: today's weight is 21 kilograms.

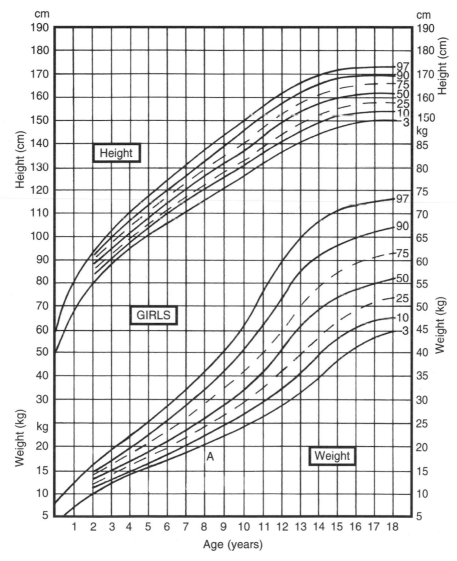

Fig. 50. Girls' age/weight curves. Courtesy Red Cliff Hospital, Red Cliff, Queensland, Australia, Dr. C. Pollard, Chief of Surgery.

Method 2

This formula is based upon age and birth weight—most mothers remember this figure because of what it did to their own figures at the time. If your child's birth weight was above or below 7 pounds you may have to extrapolate a bit, but rest assured you will get a weight upon which you can figure safe, effective drug and fluid dosages.

Example

Janie is eight years old. Consult figure 51, and apply formula (d):

$$\frac{8\,(\text{age in years})\times 7-5}{2}=25.5 \text{ kilograms}$$

One year later as you cruise the Caribbean Islands:

$$\frac{9\,(\text{age in years})\times 7-5}{2}=29 \text{ kilograms}$$

Kilograms are used because drug dosage is given in mg/kg (milligrams per kilogram) body weight. You can convert to pounds by simply multiplying kilograms by 2.2.

If you are addicted to mathematical games you will immediately uncover discrepancies between these two methods. However, either of them will give you the information you need.

When in port you may be able to weigh your child. Seek a dispensary or doctor's office—don't use a scale in a supermarket.

Weight	*Kilograms*	*(Pounds)*
(a) at birth	3.25	(7)
(b) 3–12 months	$\dfrac{\text{age}\,(\text{mo})+9}{2}$	$\left(\text{age}(\text{mo})+11\right)$
(c) 1–6 yr	$\text{age}\,(\text{yr})\times 2+8$	$\left(\text{age}(\text{yr})\times 5+17\right)$
(d) 6–12 yr	$\dfrac{\text{age}\,(\text{yr})\times 7-5}{2}$	$\left(\text{age}(\text{yr})\times 7+5\right)$
Height	*Centimeters*	*(Inches)*
(e) at birth	50	(20)
(f) at 1 yr	75	(30)
(g) 2–12 yr	$\text{age}\,(\text{yr})\times 6+77$	$\left(\text{age}(\text{yr})\times 2\frac{1}{2}+30\right)$

Fig. 51. Weight and height of normal infants and children. From *Nelson's Textbook of Pediatrics,* published by W.B. Saunders of Philadelphia.

Certain drugs are prepared in a special way for convenience in giving them to children. For example, a commercially prepared, pleasant-tasting suspension will be much easier to use than an aspirin tablet cut in two and crushed into water and sugar.

Pedialyte is a commercially prepared dry powder to mix with water and give by mouth. It is pleasant and supplies the necessary minerals to correct dehydration. If you plan to cruise in warm climates it would be well to stock up on this or similar compounds because adults too may find them more pleasant to take than salt tablets for dehydration, heat exhaustion, and similar conditions.

Figure 52 gives the generally accepted children's doses of drugs for ages up to twelve years for most situations. Certain illnesses may require different doses. These will be described in chapters devoted to discussion of these diseases.

Drug (Generic Name)	Common Name & Form	Action	Dosage & How Given
Paracetamol	Liquiprin Tylenol	analgesic antipyretic	30–40 mg/kg body wt/24 hrs; divided doses (4–6 hours by mouth)
Activated charcoal		absorbent for accidental poison ingestion	Two teaspoonsful in small glass of water
Diazepam	Valium	relief of anxiety, muscle relaxant	By mouth 0.2–0.3 mg/kg/24 hrs; divided doses every 6 hours. Watch response.
Meperidine	Demerol in single vials or larger rubber-stoppered bottle.	relief of severe pain	Deep intramuscular injection, only as necessary to control pain. Warning: Four hours after first dose, observe child's respiration and state of consciousness. If very depressed, delay the second dose for another hour. Do this with each successive dose.
Syrup of ipecac	ipecac	emetic	To induce vomiting after poison ingestion when conditions are correct. See discussion of accidental ingestion of poisons. Check package for correct dose for children.
	Lomotil (liquid, with plastic dropper)	control of diarrhea	See package insert for dosage.

Fig. 52. Drug dosage for children 2–12 years of age *(not for infants)*.

Should you wish to give a child any drug, a safe effective dose can be found by the use of Young's Rule:

$$\frac{\text{Child's weight (kilograms)}}{66} \times \text{adult dose} = \text{child's dose}$$

Example

Johnnie is eight years old and weighs 20 kg (see figure 49, age/weight curve). Dosage of said drug for an adult is 250 mg.

$$\frac{20}{66} \times 250 = 75.76$$

The dose for Johnnie is 75 mg (rounded off). This method is old, but tried and true.

As we have said, child care in advanced first aid will present difficulties not usually encountered in treating adults. The lack of history and difficulty of examination as mentioned indicate that in caring for a child you will be practicing essentially veterinary medicine. Make your best guess and go ahead. None of the remedies suggested, if used as described, will do harm and they may do a great deal of good.

The last but far from least problem you will encounter will be your own anxiety. It will likely be your own well-loved child you are forcing bad-tasting medicines upon, pricking with needles, and perhaps even sticking with rubber tubes of various kinds (catheters and/or stomach tubes). Gentleness, patience, persistence, and, above all, hiding your own anxiety from the child will greatly enhance your chances of overcoming the situation.

One final suggestion: Some medications are available in many different dosage strengths. Taking with you a supply of the proper sizes of the ones most likely needed for a young child will make treatment easier than having to cut up adult-size pills. Discuss this with your pediatrician before setting out.

CHAPTER 19

Child's Near Drowning, Ingestion of Poison, Choking, Convulsions

CHILD'S NEAR DROWNING

As in so many aspects of child care, careful attention to prevention is vital:

1. Fit the child with a life jacket that has a collar to maintain a head-up position, fits comfortably, has a strap under the crotch, and is the right size so the child will wear it. Make it a part of the child's everyday, all-the-time clothing (and night dress, if he or she gets up and wanders during the night).
2. Some may prefer that the child wear a snug harness with a tight clamp to portions of rigging. This imposes the additional responsibility of being sure it is clipped securely as the child moves about the boat.
3. Do not assume that because a child can swim he or she won't panic in the water. Many swimming-school instructors agree on this point.
4. Remember always that it takes less than ten minutes to drown. Never trust a child's judgment. You may be in the same boat of misery as the manager of the chandlery in Medang, Papua New Guinea, who left his baby daughter in the care of a nurse-maid—she went to answer the phone, was gone for five minutes, and the child drowned.

Treatment

1. Clear airway instantly no matter where the child may be.
2. Begin CPR realizing that less pressure should be used in blowing into the lungs as they can be ruptured in small children. Adjust the force used in cardiac compression as well. (Read chapter 1, "Mouth-to-Mouth Resuscitation," before you start the cruise.)
3. If there is no pulse or heartbeat begin external cardiac compression as well; continue until heartbeat and pulse are

reestablished. Read chapter 1, "Cardiac Resuscitation," before you start.

4. Keep the child's head low and be alert—often the first sign of recovery is a spasm of the diaphragm with violent vomiting of swallowed water and stomach contents. Unless the child's head is low he or she may inhale this and drown.
5. If immersion has occurred in fresh water give a single intramuscular injection of Lasix (check the package insert for dose).
6. When spontaneous breathing develops watch the patient continuously for twenty-four hours (divided watches) and be ready to resume respiratory assistance at any moment.
7. If immersion has been in filthy water, watch carefully for cough, chest pain and pus in sputum (symptoms of pneumonia), or abdominal cramps, nausea, and diarrhea (gastroenteritis symptoms). If either or both develop give antibiotics: Keflex for pneumonia, Doxycycline for gastroenteritis (one 100-mg tablet daily), both for both.
8. If the child has a period of unconsciousness and/or apnea (not breathing), evacuation to a hospital is desirable for complicated chemical studies (blood gas, O_2 CO_2), electrolytes (sodium, potassium), and blood studies (hemoglobin, protein) that can monitor the patient's recovery. But careful observation aboard your boat to assist respiration and circulation can lead to recovery, too.
9. If the child has been diving, maintain his or her head in a stable position until cervical spinal cord injury is ruled out.

Prognosis (What to Expect)

Six minutes of submersion most often has fatal results. Frequently the time underwater is not known. Don't waste time trying to find out.

If the child is conscious, gagging, choking, and/or breathing when retrieved he will recover. He needs continuous careful observation for twenty-four hours by crewpersons (divided watches) prepared to give respiratory assistance at any moment.

Voluntary gasping efforts to breathe within twenty minutes of starting resuscitation is also a very favorable sign for recovery.

If the child is unconscious and not breathing the situation is less favorable for recovery. If there is, in addition, no heartbeat, this is more unfavorable. But a few such patients with good respiratory assistance (mouth-to-mouth) and external cardiac compression have survived without brain damage.

The decision to stop resuscitation efforts is one for the heartbroken parents to make, but if there is no evidence of response after forty minutes of cardiac massage and mouth-to-mouth respiratory assistance, we would have to say that the chance for recovery is extremely remote, unless the water was very cold. See the information on hypothermia on pages 15.

Discussion

Lack of oxygen is the deadly aspect of drowning. Victims who have not aspirated (breathed) water into the lungs (10–15 percent) have better chances of recovery. The majority of these people will survive if assisted respiration is begun before the heartbeat has stopped.

Aspiration of water into the lungs causes changes in lung structures that make it hard for the sufferer to start breathing. In addition, fresh water causes changes in the surfactant substances on the lung alveoli (breathing sacs) causing many to collapse (become airless). Fresh water is hypotonic and may pass through the lung alveolar walls into the bloodstream, diluting the blood. The injection of Lasix (a diuretic) helps the kidneys to excrete this excess water.

Salt water, being hypertonic, sucks fluid from the bloodstream into the alveoli (airsacs) to partially drown out the normal CO_2/O_2 gas exchange. All these changes demand vigorous efforts when mouth-to-mouth resuscitation is given.

POISON INGESTION IN CHILDREN

The advantage to the cruising life is that the controlled environment of a boat usually prevents a child accidentally taking drugs or toxic materials. The disadvantage is that you do not have the invaluable service of the poison centers located in all major cities throughout the world. By implication then, prevention is the watchword. Certain carefully followed rules will prevent disaster:

1. All drugs and toxic products must be kept in locked cabinets.
2. Solvents or other similar materials must be stored in the original containers only.
3. No medications are to be kept in unlabelled bottles or containers and never in drink bottles.
4. A small bottle of syrup of ipecac (30 cc, one ounce) should be kept in your medicine cabinet. The use of this will be given further along.
5. All medicines and toxic substances, most of which are labelled, should have childproof tops. However, these cannot be completely depended upon.

What substances are toxic? The majority of solvents, cleaning materials, paints, paint thinners, and common medications (aspirin), as well as prescription drugs are toxic. Most substances that contain toxic material are so labelled and contain the warning "Keep out of the reach of children." Take heed.

Once ingestion has occurred there are two decisions to make:

1. Determine what the child has taken and estimate how much. This may reassure you.
2. Then decide whether to induce vomiting.

Do *not* induce vomiting when:

1. The toxin ingested is a volatile hydrocarbon such as turpentine, paint thinner, or methyl alcohol.
2. The ingested material is a strong alkali (for instance, drain cleaner). Determine this by observing the child's mouth, tongue, and lips. Strong acids and alkalies produce burns that appear as grey-white plaques on the mucous membranes.
3. The child is semiconscious or unconscious. If vomiting occurs and the child's reflexes are not active he or she may vomit, aspirate, and drown in his or her own vomit.

On the other hand *do* induce vomiting:

1. When the ingested material is some substance usually taken by mouth. These include common over-the-counter medications such as aspirin, cold tablets, or prescription drugs.
2. Three teaspoonfuls of syrup of ipecac followed by a glass of warm water will usually do the trick for a child from 1 to 12 years. For a child 6 months to 1 year, use 1 teaspoon. Do not give to a child under 6 months without advice from a health professional. You may have difficulty getting the ipecac down because it tastes bad. A poor substitute is ½ teaspoonful of table salt to a glass of water. Induce the child to swallow this. Most children will vomit within 20 minutes of taking ipecac. Ipecac is extra-effective since it empties the upper end of the small intestine as well as the stomach.

It is evident from this discussion that prevention is the sine qua non of toxic ingestion problems for small children on boats.

The follow-up treatment available for accidental ingestion on a cruising vessel is similar regardless of the substance ingested.

1. Maintain adequate respiration; keep the airway open. Remove all foreign material from the mouth; be sure the tongue is not swallowed. Keep the child lying on his or her left side, head lower than hips, and neck extended; suction mucus from mouth

and throat by using your own mouth suction through a small plastic tube. Keep the lungs clear by encouraging the patient to cough; roll him or her back and forth to help clear the lungs. Mouth-to-mouth breathing assistance may be needed.

2. Reduce the absorption of substances already swallowed:
   a. Make a mixture of 1 or 2 teaspoonfuls of flavored activated charcoal in a small glass of water and encourage the child to drink it. The charcoal will absorb and inactivate many poisons, allowing them to progress harmlessly through the bowels.
   b. When conditions are proper—as described previously—induce vomiting by administration of three teaspoonfuls of syrup of ipecac in a glass of warm water. Disregard the child's objection to the foul taste.
3. Keep the child well supplied with favorite drinks to increase drug excretion by the kidneys.

Drugs and Household Materials Most Commonly Taken by Children
Based on the experience of emergency rooms of major hospitals, the following drugs and compounds, many of which are easily accessible, are those most commonly taken accidentally by children.
Aspirin. A common ingestion. It is available and most baby aspirin preparations have a pleasant flavor.
   Dangerous dose. Ages three to six years: 250–300 mg/kg of body weight.
   Action. On the brain, especially on the breathing and heat control centers.
   Symptoms. Increase in rate and depth of breathing, vomiting, confusion, buzzing in the ears, elevated temperature, coma.
   Treatment. If the child is alert and responsive, induce vomiting. If he or she is drowsy or unconscious, support breathing only (see above).
Paracetamol. Many painkilling preparations—Panadol, etc.
   Dangerous dose. Varies greatly but 10 gm can be fatal in the young.
   Action. Produces liver damage in three to four days.
   Treatment. Induce vomiting at once. Keep the child hydrated by oral drinks (water, Coke, etc.).
Strong Alkalies. Drain-cleaning compounds, lye, etc.
   Action. Strong alkali produces burns, wherever it touches, that appear as greyish plaques on mouth, face, tongue, and lips.
   Symptoms. Severe pain, nausea, and salivation (excess production of spit). If burns of the throat are severe (depends upon amount swallowed), this will produce chest or upper back pain, inability to swallow, and severe drooling of saliva.

Treatment. Do not induce vomiting—acid in the stomach will neutralize the alkali. Vomiting merely raises the material back into the esophagus and throat to cause more burns. After neutralization by stomach acid the alkali will pass harmlessly through the gastrointestinal tract. Wash all visible burns with copious amounts of water. Give pain medication (Demerol) according to Young's Rule. If severe symptoms of esophageal burns appear (see above), evacuation is urgent. Esophagoscopy is needed.

Barbiturates. Usually taken by older children—sleeping pills, Nembutal, Seconal, Phenobarbital, etc.

Dangerous dose. 1 gm; 3 gm is potentially lethal.

Action. Depresses brain function, especially the breathing center.

Symptoms. Grade I: drowsy but responds to verbal communications. Grade II: unconscious but responds to minimal stimulation. Grade III: unconscious but responds to maximal painful stimulations. Grade IV: unconscious, no response to maximal stimulation. Stimulation: rubbing sternum (breastbone) with rolled-up fist.

Treatment. Sustain breathing, mouth-to-mouth if necessary. Do not induce vomiting if the child is drowsy. Sustain respiration only. Keep supplied with drinks to keep the kidneys functioning to eliminate the poison from the body. Give charcoal slurry if the child can swallow.

Hydrocarbons. Petroleum ether, naptha, gasoline, kerosene, turpentine, fuel oil, mineral seal oil. Ninety percent of the ingestions of these occur in children under five years of age.

Dangerous dose. Any amount, but half an ounce has caused death.

Action. Main harm is from fumes inhaled or liquid content spilled into the lung as these pass the laryngeal opening on the way down the esophagus to the stomach. Inflammation of the lung (pneumonitis) is immediate and may lead to severe pneumonia in hours or days, depending on the amount that gets into the lungs.

Symptoms. Severe lung irritation, cough, and respiratory distress. Diarrhea may follow in a few hours or days.

Treatment. Main effort is to assure that adequate lung ventilation is maintained. Keep airway clear, suck out any obstructing mucus. If increasing chest pain and fever suggest pneumonia, particularly if pus is coughed up, then antibiotics of proper dosage —see chapter 18—should be given. Initiating vomiting is *not* advised.

CHOKING

The young child is busy exploring this new world into which he has been somewhat forcefully thrust. Much of this adventure is via the mouth. Note how frequently a small child pops anything and everything into his mouth. There is always the possibility of swallowing or inhaling a small solid object. Don't have any on board. No peanuts or popcorn-type snacks, or toys that easily come apart into small pieces.

Swallowed objects are usually not dangerous. It is axiomatic that almost anything a child can swallow will go on through the stomach, the small and large intestine, and emerge at the other end. Keep a sharp lookout for it for a few days.

A solid object which is inhaled or stuck in the oropharynx will cause varying amounts of choking and respiratory distress. You will have to try to remove the foreign body. Do not employ mouth-to-mouth respiration until you get the foreign body out or you may drive it more firmly into place.

The Heimlich maneuver (see "Café Coronary Disease," chapter 12) should be tried. Another method is to place the child face down across your knees with mouth down and thump him on the back till the obstruction pops out. Efforts to reach down through the mouth with your fingers will usually be futile, but may be attempted if all else fails.

A foreign body inhaled into the trachea (windpipe) can cause cough, hoarseness, dyspnea (difficult breathing), and asthmatic wheezing. The method of attempted removal is as described above.

If a small child has a violent coughing and choking attack which subsides after a few hours or a day or two and no foreign body is coughed up, this is a matter of concern. What may have happened is that a small foreign body (peanut, tooth, etc.) has lodged deep in the bronchus (lung tube) and irritation due to its presence has subsided. However, a visit to medical facilities at the next major port should be made for X-ray and other examinations to be sure that no foreign body is present. If there is, it must be removed by bronchoscopy because if left it may cause a lung abscess many weeks, or even months, after the original incident.

CONVULSIONS

A convulsion, which is described as a violent contraction of all the muscles of the child's body, usually with a loss of consciousness, is the most alarming symptom to child and parent that can be imagined. Generally speaking there are two types of convulsions, but there are many different causes of convulsions.

The first type of convulsion is fairly common among children who suffer a fever. Particularly if the fever comes on rather rapidly and is high, somewhere along the line the child may have a severe generalized convulsion. The seizures occurring with sudden onset of high fever are treated by controlling the infectious disease that has caused the high fever. If it is a bacterial infection it will be, of course, with antibiotics. If it is a viral infection, there is no specific management.

The other type of convulsion is due to some underlying brain disease or brain malfunction. This second type needs thorough hospital and neurosurgical examination.

The management of the actual convulsion (seizure) itself is, in spite of its alarming manifestations, not very complicated. The child should be secured to avoid injury. Some advise placing a soft balled-up towel or something of this nature into the mouth so the chattering teeth won't chew the tongue to ribbons. Valium by intravenous route is most efficacious in treating convulsions. Please check the package insert very carefully. If no one is able to administer the drug intravenously, then intramuscular administration of Valium should be considered.

CHAPTER 20

Childhood Appendicitis (Special Problems), Pinworms

ACUTE APPENDICITIS

This, the most common abdominal surgical disease, may occur at any age from a few days to eighty or more years. It is more common in young to middle-aged persons. Certain aspects of the disease in children deserve discussion. The diagnosis is more difficult in inverse ratio to the child's age: the very young cannot tell you where it hurts, they localize tenderness poorly, and so can furnish little useful history or observations upon abdominal examination. If you are lucky, are a patient parent, and have a cooperative child up to the age of six or seven years, there is one maneuver that may help you to a diagnosis when acute appendicitis is suspected.

This is the rectal examination. As shown in figure 53, it is possible, if managed properly, to place your examining finger quite close to the appendix. If it is inflamed it will be tender to the touch through the rectal wall. Should you approach your child, an out-thrust finger dripping with Vaseline and a grim look on your face, you will likely encourage the child to resist with or without screaming and defeat the attempt. So try it this way.

Rectal Examination of a Child

1. One-half hour before the attempt, give the child a sedative, with dosage according to Young's Rule.
2. Have the child lie down on his or her back on a bunk or, better, across mother's lap, knees drawn up.
3. Hold the child firmly but gently. Do not grab or clutch.
4. Gently spread the buttocks.
5. Place well-lubricated (with Vaseline, salad oil, etc.) tip of first finger (right or left according to your handedness) just at the outer margin of the anus. Apply gentle steady pressure.
6. When the fuss from this subsides, rotate the finger and pass through the anal muscle ring with a circular motion.

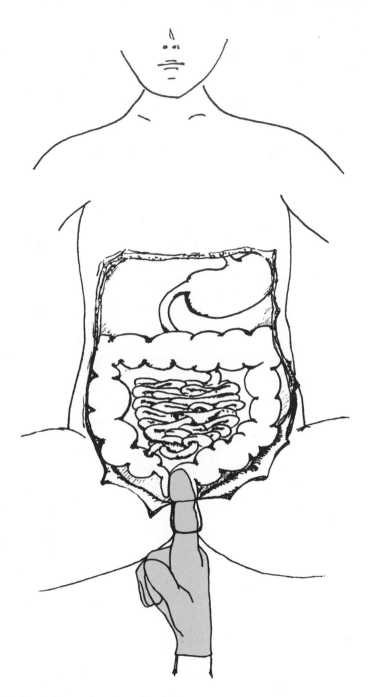

Fig. 53. Rectal examination of a child.

7. When the fussing subsides again, slowly advance the finger as far as it goes easily.
8. Press fingertip against rectal wall to the left (this is the side away from the appendix). It should not be painful if you are slow and gentle.
9. Slowly turn fingertip and press right side of upper rectal wall. If the appendix is inflamed, this will be painful. Such a finding strongly suggests acute appendicitis. Unfortunately the appendix may be in another location, so a negative finding must be interpreted with caution.
10. Slowly withdraw finger and comfort the child.

Your finesse, skill, and gentleness, plus a huge dollop of luck, may prevent the onset of indignant screams from the outset and so facilitate the examination.

There is no objection to giving a low enema or a suppository to a child when attempting to discover if the abdominal pain is due to constipation, but *never* give a laxative. This may cause an infected appendix to rupture.

PINWORMS

If you are a lover not only of children but also of animals, and you take a dog or cat cruising with children, have them all dewormed before you take off (pets and the whole family). Pinworms, which 90 percent of dog owners enjoy together with their pets, may be a cause of acute appendicitis. Worms get down into the appendix, ulcerate the mucosal lining, and start off the infection. Not all physicians agree, but the author has seen this happen.

CHAPTER 21

Treatment of a Severely Burned Child (Special Problems), Dehydration

Prevention of a large burn is worth whatever efforts it demands:

1. Keep matches and cigarette lighters locked up all the time.
2. Stow all inflammables in locked cabinets above decks (gasoline, kerosene, methylated spirits, etc.).
3. Leave no food cooking on the stove unwatched.
4. Recognize that water heated by passage through the boat's diesel engine heat exchanger may be hot enough to scald a child.
5. Know intimately the location of fire extinguishers and keep them uncluttered.

Burns can vary from a mild annoyance to a life-threatening, horrible injury. The severity of the burn depends upon the depth of the burn and the percentage of the body area involved.

Depth of Burn

1. First degree: skin reddened only; rarely dangerous, unless total body sunburn.
2. Second degree: blisters, destruction of upper layers of skin. Sensitive to pinprick. Will heal without scarring if infection is prevented.
3. Third degree: complete destruction of all layers of skin and at times underlying structures. If over an inch in diameter, will not heal without skin grafting.

See color plate in chapter 4 opposite page 76.

Percentage of Body Area Burned
An adult follows the Rule of Nines. *A child does not.* Figure 54 shows percentage variation of body surface area for ages one to twelve years. Any burn of more than 10 percent of body surface or second or third

degree is a serious injury. Burn shock may develop in the first twenty-four hours following injury. This condition is described in chapter 4.

Should a child suffer a severe burn it will be extremely upsetting to both victim and entire crew. Best have a plan to manage the situation:

1. *Put out the fire on the child's clothes or body instantly.* Roll the child on the deck, douse with a bucket of water, or drop overside if at anchor in reasonably clean water. Don't wait to remove clothes. The severity of burn is determined by heat plus contact as measured in seconds of exposure.
2. Assess other injuries if there has been an explosion. Be sure airway is clear if face is involved.
3. Sedate the child with a proper dose of Demerol by injection. Use Young's Rule:

$$\frac{\text{Child's weight (lbs)}}{150} \times \text{adult dose} = \text{child's dose}$$

Lay the child on a clean sheet in good work space.
4. Cool all burns with moist compresses. Place fresh- or seawater or ice over a compress for three to five minutes only.
5. Make a careful estimate of the depth of burns and body surface involved. If more than 10 percent of the body surface is burned to the second or third degree you have a serious injury to care for. Burn shock is not apparent immediately, but develops in the first twelve to twenty-four hours post-burn.

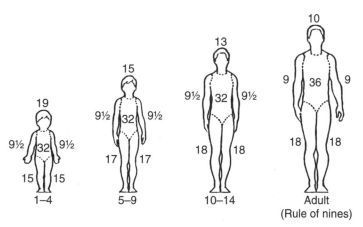

Fig. 54. Burn assessment chart. Bold numbers under the figures indicate age; the others indicate percent of body surface. From *Nelson's Textbook of Pediatrics,* published by W.B. Saunders, Philadelphia.

6. Boil for twenty minutes two quarts of fresh water in a covered pan containing a small pair of scissors and tweezers (any type—the kind for plucking eyebrows will do). Allow to cool.
7. Scrub your hands for five minutes with Betadine and fresh water; clean your fingernails. Put on sterile gloves.
8. Clean up the wound. Cut away with scissors any loose skin, burned clothing, etc. Anything that comes away easily should be removed. Then scrub area gently with gauze pad and detergent. *Do not rupture or disturb intact blisters.*
9. Rinse thoroughly with boiled cooled water. Pat dry with gauze or a clean towel.
10. When debridement (which you have just done) is complete, move the child to a bunk on a clean sheet or towel.
11. Apply generous amounts of Silvadene 1%. Dress the burn with sterile gauze squares or cut-up clean towels, sheets, rags, etc.
12. Apply a pressure dressing—Ace bandages or KLING wrapped about the limb or body—firmly, but not tightly enough to stop circulation.

The onset of burn shock in the child will present symptoms of weakness, pallor, sweating, and diminishing urine output. The loss of fluids into the burned area diminishes the circulating blood volume which slows urine output. Similarly, if you are treating burn shock as about to be described, you can measure your success by improving symptoms which are often preceded by increasing urinary output.

1. Pass a catheter and leave in-lying (see chapter 6). Calculate the child's fluid needs for the first twenty-four hours.
2. The urine output as collected by catheter and measured will furnish the best information to anticipate the onset of burn shock, even before weakness, sweating, rapid pulse, and other symptoms are evident (see chapter 4).

Normal Hourly Urine Output by Age

3–5 yrs	6–8 yrs	9–10 yrs	10–12 yrs
8cc/hr	12cc/hr	24cc/hr	24cc/hr

If urine output drops below these normals, burn shock is likely on the way. After the administration of parenteral (injected) fluid (see chapter 4) or drinks (with no vomiting), if the urine output rises to normal this indicates recovery from burn shock. If urine output remains normal following a burn this indicates absence of burn shock (which is rare in an extensive burn, i.e., more than 15 percent of body surface of second- or third-degree burn).

Fluid requirements for the first twenty-four hours following a severe burn are arrived at by adding together two separate requirements:

1. Normal maintenance that a healthy child would need anyway (sweating, vaporizing lung air, urine).
2. Extra fluid because of loss of fluid seeping from burned areas and swelling of parts around burned area.

Normal Daily Maintenance for Losses Due to Diarrhea or Vomiting
120 cc per kilogram up to 1,000 cc in first year of life, plus 100 cc for each additional year of life.

Example 1
An eight-year-old boy with a body weight of 20 kilograms (see age/weight curves in figure 49):

1,000 cc for first year of life	1,000
100 cc for each additional year of life (100 × 7)	700
Total daily requirements for loss due to seasickness, diarrhea, or vomiting	1,700 cc

1,700 cc equals 1 quart (1,000 cc) plus 1 pint (500 cc) plus 200 cc in 24 hours.

Extra Fluid Requirement for Burns

Example 2
Same child with a 20 percent body burn (20 percent of second or third degree) requires the above normal (1,700 cc) plus, for burn:

$$\frac{\% \text{ of body area burned} \times \text{body weight in kilograms}}{2}$$

$$\frac{20\% \times 8 \text{ kg}}{2} = \frac{1.6}{2} = .8 \text{ liter} = \quad \frac{800 \text{ cc}}{2,500 \text{ cc}}$$

2,500 cc equals 2 quarts (2,000 cc) plus 1 pint (500 cc).

These are standard formulas from the Royal Children's Hospital of Queensland University Department of Child Care. These figures vary with the age of the child.

This is a considerable quantity of fluid to give by subcutaneous injection. It will swell the areas into which it is injected but, since it is not given intravenously, will not overload the heart and lungs.

You can estimate your success—if the urine output has been below normal and is rising toward normal you are treating the burn shock successfully. If this is not taking place, change the site of fluid injection and keep at it.

Fluid Requirements for the Second Twenty-Four Hours Following a Major Burn

1. Normal maintenance according to Example 1, above.
2. If urine output is normal or rising toward normal (see page 196), add half the additional fluid for burn (Example 2).
3. If urine output is not normal or not rising, repeat the original amount calculated in Example 2, above. Subtract any fluids taken by mouth.
4. If the child is vomiting, estimate the amount lost and add an equal amount of normal saline to the fluids injected.

By the third day, the child could be recovering and able to take fluids by mouth. Small sips of milk or fruit juice at frequent intervals are often tolerated, even though the child is nauseated and vomiting occasionally. Start to feed a high-calorie, high-protein diet as soon as tolerated. As more fluid is drunk, reduce subcutaneous fluid injection proportionally.

The intravenous method used by doctors, nurses, and paramedics allows faster administration and additional protein-containing fluids to be given. The subcutaneous method is slower and only normal saline solution (salt and water) can be given. However, it is simple (it can be learned by anyone in five minutes—see chapter 4) and easier to maintain on a cruising vessel. It will do the best job possible.

To prepare fluids for subcutaneous injection:

1. Measure correct amount of fresh water in a graduated liter cylinder. Add the proper number of salt tablets (as marked on the bottle) to make normal saline. *Keep salt tablets in a tightly stoppered container except when actually removing some.*
2. Boil water for five minutes; allow to cool.
3. Start subcutaneous fluid injection or 5% DRL—1,000 cc with tubing and needles. If there is some fluid left over, keep it in a covered container until you can put the rest in the sterile bottle. *Do not use salt solution made more than twenty-four hours prior to use. Discard it and make fresh.* Use only if you don't have 5% DRL.
4. Dressings should be changed as necessary, i.e., when dirty, wet, and smelly. Sedate the child half an hour before you remove the dressings. Wash the burns with boiled cooled water and detergents. Apply antibacterial ointment. Old dressings can be washed, dried, and reused when clean.

5. High fever (101–102° F), together with increasing redness and swelling of burn areas, demands that systemic antibiotics in proper dosage be given; Keflex by mouth is preferable, but, if the child is vomiting, use injectable Rocephin.
6. Sedatives may be given as needed in the following hours and days.

It is obvious from the complexity of management that evacuation of a severely burned child as soon as possible is advisable.

Discussion

Extensive burns are serious injuries. Losses of fluids (protein, electrolytes, blood, water) are tremendous into burned and surrounding areas. Evaporation of fluid from the burned surface also contributes to the loss. The administration of various fluids (amino acids, blood, protein hydrolysates, albumen, and other complex combinations) is the subject of much discussion among physicians who care for burns in hospitals. However, there is not much argument that the administration of normal saline solution is helpful—perhaps, from some studies, most helpful. And this is something that you can do for a burned child on board your boat. You may find it difficult to give the total fluid amounts suggested by the subcutaneous route. These will cause swelling of the area into which they are injected but will ultimately be absorbed.

Often a burn appears more horrible than it really is. For instance, a second-degree burn of 8 percent of body surface (a child's chest) will blister and look horrible. If cleaned up and dressed to prevent infection it will heal without scarring in a couple of weeks. Such a healed burn does not tolerate exposure to sunlight well.

Long-term follow-up care of an extensive burn calls for professional medical treatment and often hospitalization. If it is a third-degree burn, skin grafts will be needed. Psychiatric help will be necessary to overcome the severe emotional trauma that accompanies an extensive burn. The parents will probably need emotional help, too, because, regardless of the circumstances at the time of injury, they will most often have a heavy burden of guilt.

DEHYDRATION

Any illness which causes fluid loss because of diminished intake, vomiting, diarrhea, bleeding, or excessive sweating (see chapter 5, "Heat Exhaustion") may cause dehydration (loss of circulating blood volume). Because the child needs a daily exchange rate of 25 percent of total fluids (adults need 9 percent by comparison) serious dehydration develops rapidly.

You must be familiar with signs and symptoms of dehydration of your sick or injured child, whatever the cause. See figure 55.

Fluid replacement is best by mouth. If the child is eating, food will replace the necessary chemicals lost.

If the child is not eating, but can retain fluids, the druggist has a selection of flavored powders that contain the necessary electrolytes. Stock some in your first aid kit. Simply add these to water as directed and encourage the child to drink. If you have none available, salty lemonade can be made from a teaspoonful of salt to a quart of water with any available flavoring. This will be less pleasant than the prepared powders but will do the job. It may be nauseating. Use less salt.

If a child is vomiting occasionally it may be possible to maintain hydration with small sips of prepared solutions, salty lemonade, or

Signs and Symptoms	Mild	Moderate	Severe
General appearance and condition in infants and young children	Thirsty, alert, restless	Thirsty, restless or lethargic but irritable to touch or drowsy	Drowsy, limp, cold, sweaty; extremities blue; may be comatose
Older children and adults	Thirsty, alert, restless	Thirsty, alert; postural hypotension (faint on standing erect)	Usually conscious; apprehensive, cold, sweaty, cyanotic; extremities (fingers, toes) wrinkled skin; muscle cramps
Radial pulse (at wrist)	Normal rate and volume	Rapid, weak	Rapid, feeble, sometimes impalpable
Respiration	Normal	Deep, may be rapid, normal, or low	Deep and rapid
Systolic blood pressure	Normal	Normal or low	Less than 90 mm/Hg; may be unrecordable
Skin elasticity	Pinch retracts immediately	Pinch retracts slowly	Pinch retracts very slowly, 2 seconds or longer
Eyes	Normal	Sunken (detectably)	Grossly sunken
Tears	Present	Absent	Very dry eyes
Membranes (mucous)	Moist	Dry	Very dry
Urine flow	Normal	Reduced amount; dark	None passed for several hours; empty bladder

Fig. 55. Clinical assessment of severity of dehydration. From *Nelson's Textbook of Pediatrics* by permission of W.B. Saunders, Inc., of Philadelphia.

milk. Sufficient fluid may be retained. You can judge this by watching for development of the signs and symptoms described in figure 55.

If the child is vomiting or losing fluid from severe diarrhea, you will have to give fluids by parenteral means. At sea this means intravenous or subcutaneous injection of normal salt solution, as described earlier in this chapter. Normal saline is the only fluid you can give, but fortunately it supplies a most essential chemical element—sodium. Don't be afraid to use it or 5% DRL.

If giving fluids to replace losses from diarrhea or vomiting, you will give *only the normal daily requirements* described earlier in this chapter and not the much larger amounts required in the treatment of burns.

Seasickness
This may be a cause for serious dehydration and may require parenteral fluids in amounts similar to those for burns. For seasickness use various remedies in reduced dosage. Young's Rule may be used:

$$\frac{\text{Child's weight (pounds)}}{150} \times \text{adult dose} = \text{child's dose}$$

CHAPTER 22

Bacterial Meningitis

Daniel, thirty-five-year-old skipper of *Sun Seeker,* a 36-foot cruising ketch, sat alone in the cockpit with a list in his hand. The last, he hoped, of several hundred he had worked through in the past six months.

The boat had been beefed up for ocean cruising. Will, his six-year-old son, protesting loudly, had had his immunizations brought up to date by his pediatrician. Daniel and Janie, his thirty-four-year-old wife, had seen their family physician, who, after consultation with the San Diego Health Department, advised inoculations for tetanus, typhoid and paratyphoid, and cholera.

Farewell parties over the past week had been tiring but soon they would be away from such social pressures. Midafternoon, Janie and Will came aboard, having attended a party at Will's preschool group in honor of his departure. They had a quiet dinner at the San Diego Yacht Club and went early to bed for a bright and early start.

9 March: Weather reports from Point Loma were favorable and they shoved off.

12 March: GPS showed they were some 325 miles on their way. They had all sailed a lot before, Will since the age of two and a half, so they got their sea legs on in a hurry.

14 March: Will awoke with symptoms of a cold. Janie noted:

1. Nose red and swollen,
2. Eyes reddened,
3. Throat red and scratchy,
4. A dry, tight cough, nonproductive.

He must have caught something at the school party, she thought. She gave him aspirin dosage according to Young's Rule and did her best to keep him quiet. It was difficult—he was so excited. Will's symptoms subsided over the next three days but he didn't really recover completely. No fever daily, but somewhat listless behavior, which was unusual for him.

18 March: Nine days on the way, approaching the doldrums: 12° south latitude, 138° west longitude, wind becoming fluky, thunderstorms around the horizon. Will woke up with a headache, felt weak and sick. Janie hoped he hadn't got the flu. She gave him aspirin and kept him quiet in his bunk. He was willing to stay quiet. His headache got worse during the day. Daniel took his temperature at dusk, 101.8°F. During the night Will complained of his head "hurting more." Janie noted:

1. Weakness and prostration.
2. Vomiting in projectile fashion at midnight.
3. At dawn headache worse, vomited several times.
4. Complained of light hurting his eyes (photophobia).
5. Very reluctant to raise head or bend neck (meningismus).
6. Janie raised his head to give him a drink. His legs bent sharply at the knees—she couldn't straighten them out.
7. Temperature 103°F.
8. Difficult to arouse, more deeply asleep.

Janie had a look at the child-sized sketch inside the back cover of her first aid manual. Will had symptoms of bacterial meningitis.

TREATMENT

To treat Will, Janie gave him Rocephin by deep intramuscular injection with calculated pediatric dose.

By next afternoon, twelve hours after the first injection of Rocephin, Will appeared better:

1. His headache was less painful.
2. He was more alert—able to carry out verbal commands.
3. His temperature was down to 100°F.
4. There was no vomiting—he took sips of fluid by mouth.
5. His neck hurt less.

Janie gave the second day's dose of Rocephin by injection. On the following morning—forty-eight hours after beginning treatment—Will was definitely better:

1. His headache was almost gone.
2. His neck was no longer stiff.
3. He was alert and responsive.
4. His temperature was 99°F.

Three days after onset, Will was alert, responding, and complaining only of his sore bottom:

1. His headache was gone.
2. His neck wasn't stiff.
3. He was very alert and responsive.
4. His temperature read 98.6°F at 1900.

Four days after onset, Will was afebrile (without fever) and hungry. Janie stopped the injections, but continued medicating by using Cipro in divided doses daily on a calculated pediatric dose, until she had completed a total of ten days' treatment. Will found it easy to swallow those big pills as long as no one came in his direction with those awful needles. Of course Janie's courage and the needles had saved his life.

Discussion

Bacterial meningitis is an infectious disease which attacks children and, less often, adults. It is caused by any one of a number of bacteria: *Neisseria meningitidis, Haemophilus influenzae, Diplococcus pneumoniae, Escherichia coli,* or *Staphylococcus aureus.* It is transmitted by contact from an infected person.

When the bacteria takes over, pus forms on the meninges or membranes lining the brain and spinal canal. The onset can be swift and devastating. The child becomes desperately ill in a matter of hours. Some days before the disease develops there is often what appears to be an upper respiratory infection. This is the time when the bacteria are entering the body through the upper respiratory passages. The stiff neck and reflex flexion of the legs (Brudzinski's sign) and resistance to straightening them (Kernig's sign) are diagnostic. Before the days of antibiotic treatment, nine out of ten children who contracted bacterial meningitis died. The few who survived were often totally deaf or mentally retarded. Modern antibiotic treatment, given early, has changed this a great deal.

Fortunately Janie had done her homework—recognized the onset of the condition early and began intensive antibiotic therapy. She knew that intravenous therapy was desirable and if there had been a hospital nearby, a spinal puncture to find certain changes in the spinal fluid would have established a diagnosis. These modes were not available to her so she bravely did the best she could. It proved lifesaving to little Will. She knew a virus may cause meningitis, in which case the antibiotic treatment would be useless. But luck, if anything in such a desperate situation can be called luck, was on her side. If the response to Rocephin had not been satisfactory, she could have added a second antibiotic such as Keflex or Cipro by mouth (see chapter 7).

Early, not panic-stricken, but careful attention to fever, stiff neck, positive Brudzinski's and Kernig's signs will establish the early diagnosis. Antibiotic treatment is most effective at this stage of the disease.

CHAPTER 23

Bacillary Dysentery
(Shigellosis)

Dora and Ralph, first mate and skipper of *Jolly Roger,* a 36-foot sailing ketch, together with their eight-year-old daughter, Robin, enjoyed their visit to Wallis Island in the western Pacific. The night before departing for Tonga they had dinner at the concrete shed café on the pier. It was primitive: dogs, pigs, and children filtered through the doorless front entrance to wander around the dining tables; the floor was packed earth; the tables were rough planks covered with linoleum laid on sawhorses.

The food was exquisite: a seafood bisque followed by broiled lobster, crumbed fish, vegetables, a bottle of good white wine, and a sweet at the end. The bill was a shock—just what they would pay in a luxury restaurant with more civilized accommodations.

Twenty-four hours underway to Tonga they ran into a flat calm. They had gotten no extra fuel in Wallis Island so they drifted. Dora and Robin complained of pain—vague, "all over" the abdomen. They lost their appetite.

Next morning both stomachaches were worse and young Robin looked flushed, anxious, and sick. During the day the youngster complained of increasing abdominal pain and had one loose runny bowel movement every hour accompanied by cramping pain. Her mother had some loose stools, but no cramps.

Young Robin turned into her bunk at dusk but got up every hour to perch on the head, passing loose stools and groaning with cramps.

Ralph examined her when she got off her perch:

1. Her face was flushed, her expression anxious. She was sweating and pale. Her oral temperature was 40°C (104°F).
2. Her pulse was 120 per minute.
3. Her abdomen was gurgling, tender all over to gentle palpation.
4. He flashed a light into the head—her last stool was runny, thin, and streaked with mucus and red blood.

A look at the child's diagnostic chart in the back of his first aid book found that for diarrhea, mucus and blood in the stool, and fever, the diagnosis is bacillary dysentery.

I guess we aren't through paying for that fancy dinner yet, he thought.

TREATMENT

1. Since fluid loss from diarrhea may be tremendous, the patients were urged to increase their usual fluid intake. If the diarrhea continues to be severe the "salty lemonade" is an excellent replacement for the lost fluids and electrolytes.
2. Once the decision has been made that this is more than a simple diarrhea—i.e., fever, severe abdominal cramps with the stool streaked with blood and mucus, antibiotics are in order.

The adult dose for Bactrim DS is one tablet twice daily. Since Robin weighs only 27 kg, one-half of the adult dose is sufficient.

In adults (over 18 years of age), Cipro 500 mg twice daily is very effective as an alternative. A course of any of the antibiotics available on board should be continued for a minimum of five days.

3. A hot-water bottle helps relieve abdominal discomfort.
4. Lomotil should be *avoided* in a bacterial diarrhea as it slows down the transit time of the bacteria-laden stool and may prolong the febrile state.

Ralph gave mother Dora:

1. Cipro 500 mg two times a day.
2. A Lomotil tablet after each loose bowel movement since she did not have fever or mucus and blood in the stool. Using up to eight tablets per day may be very helpful for any adult in a non-bacterial diarrhea. Approximately half these doses can be used in children.

Next morning both patients were improved. The wind finally came up and when they arrived at Vau Vau in Tonga three days later all were well and happy.

Discussion
Bacillary dysentery is distributed worldwide. It is caused by the Salmonella group of bacteria. Feces-to-mouth transmission by unclean hands and dishes is the usual method of transmission. Someone may

have an acute attack and recover without the use of antibiotics, but then often becomes a carrier of the disease.

Ralph weighed his daughter at every opportunity—a wise precaution because drug dosage and fluid needs in sick or hurt children are determined by body weight. Most cruising vessels probably won't bring along a scale capable of weighing a child.

Figures 49, 50, and 51, in chapter 18, present two methods of computing a child's weight. Neither is as accurate as a proper scale but will give close enough poundage for safe, effective drug dosage.

Ralph replaced Robin's fluid and electrolyte losses by giving her salty lemonade to drink: one quart of water, one level teaspoonful salt flavored with lemon. If he had purchased prior to departure Pedialyte or any of a number of packaged, flavored electrolyte powders to be added to water, he would have had Robin drink this. Her thirst plus her urine output would be the best guide to determine how much fluid she would need.

Glossary

Limited definition of terms as used in medical practice.

Acid chyme. Mixture of food, hydrochloric acid, and pepsin and rennin enzymes fashioned in the stomach during digestion of food.

Anaphylaxis. Severe collapse that occurs when an individual is challenged by a food or drug to which he or she is highly allergic. Can be fatal.

Antibacterial. Any substance harmful to bacteria.

Antibody. Immune substance produced in the living body when it is challenged by a foreign protein.

Antiemetic. Drugs or substances to stop or prevent vomiting.

Arm. Upper extremity from elbow to shoulder.

Asepsis. The technique of making a wound sterile by removing or destroying all bacteria.

Aspiration. Inhaling fluids or solids into the lungs. Occurs when a patient is unconscious and gag and cough reflexes are depressed.

Bedsores. Weak or paralyzed patients may lie too long on one spot, squeezing the blood from it; the tissue dies and falls away leaving an open sore.

B.i.d. Two times daily.

Bilirubin. Bile pigment derived from hemoglobin breakdown.

Bilirubinuria. Excess bile in urine. Makes urine an orange color—accompanies jaundice.

Boardlike abdomen. Rigid abdomen that feels as hard as a table. Accompanies perforated ulcer of the duodenum or other viscus (organ).

Bowel obstruction. Blockage of flow of bowels. May be mechanical (as with impaction) or reflex (as in peritonitis, from interruption of nerve impulses).

Bulb syringe. Wide glass barrel with rubber bulb. Similar to a douche syringe or a turkey baster.

Butterflies. Adhesive tape bridges to close a wound.

Chemotherapeutic. Chemical agents (sulfa drugs and related compounds) that have antibacterial action.

Clitoris. Female analogy of male penis.

Coma. Loss of conscious response. Varies in degree and duration. Caused by blows, infections, or severe imbalance of body chemistry, as diabetic coma.

Cubic centimeter. Fluid volume measure. One one-thousandth of a liter.

Duodenum. First 12 inches of the small intestine.

Enteric-coated. Outer coating for pill that will dissolve in the small intestine rather than in the stomach (e.g., salt pill).

Enzymes. Substances that are necessary for a chemical reaction but do not change character as a result of such reactions.

External cardiac compression. Technique of putting pressure on the chest (with the patient lying on the back) to cause blood to be squeezed out of the heart and to flow through the arteries to the brain and vital structures when normal heartbeat has stopped temporarily.

Fibroblasts. Young connective tissue cells that mature into scar.

Flaccid paralysis. Completely limp paralysis, usually of an extremity. Often seen in head injury and stroke with unconsciousness.

Foley catheter. Rubber tube inserted into the urinary bladder when patient is unable to void. This type has a small balloon on the inner end which can be inflated to hold the catheter in the bladder.

Forearm. Upper extremity from wrist to elbow.

Fracture. Broken bone.
Simple. Broken bone, unbroken skin.
Compound. Skin overlying broken bone is broken.

Genitourinary tract. Urinary tract (*q.v.*) plus genitals: In the male, penis and testes. In the female, ovaries, fallopian tubes, uterus, clitoris, labia, and vagina.

Gram. Metric measure of weight. One gram equals the weight of one cubic centimeter of water under standard conditions.

Great omentum. A fold of peritoneal (abdominal lining) membrane that swings free from the lower edge of the stomach. It is known as "the abdominal policeman" because it is somewhat mobile and hastens to the site of a perforation or infection in an abdominal organ and seals it off.

Groin. Crease between the lower abdomen and upper thigh.

Healing by first intention. Primary healing of a wound without infection or delay.

Healing by second intention. Healing of a wound which has been infected and/or separated and must fill in with scar tissue.

Hematoma. A blood clot in the body tissues.

Hemostatic mechanism. Those body organ systems that keep internal environment (temperature, acid/base balance, fluid volumes) quite constant despite varying demands from the environment.

H.S. Hour of sleep.

Hypothermia. A lowering of core body temperature by immersion in cold water or air, causing the patient to appear to be dead: no movement, no breathing, no palpable pulse. Resuscitation may be possible if the condition is recognized.

Jaundice. Yellow color of skin and eyeballs due to retention of bile in the system.

Leg. Lower extremity from ankle to knee.

Leucocytes. White blood cells.

Liter. Metric measure of liquid. Approximately equal to 1 quart.

Lymphadenitis. Swelling of lymph nodes at knee, groin, elbow, armpit, or neck, indicating that infection beyond is extending toward the bloodstream.

Lymphangitis. Red streaks extending out from a wound or

infection, indicating that infection is spreading toward the bloodstream from the site.

Lymph node. Nodule of filtering tissue in the lymphatic fluid system.

Metabolism. The sum total of chemical activity in the living body.

Milligram. Metric measure of solids. 1/1000 gram. Many potent drugs are measured in milligrams (mg).

Milliliter. One one-thousandth of a liter—liquid measure. See Cubic Centimeter.

Mittelschmerz. Middle sickness. Abdominal pain in women due to a small amount of blood spilling from the ovary at the time of ovulation, usually in mid-menstrual cycle. Hence the name.

Nasogastric tube. A rubber or plastic tube for insertion through the nose down the gullet, and into the stomach. Suitably marked to indicate when it is in the stomach, it is used for emptying or filling the stomach.

Near-drowning. Survival after near fatal submersion in water.

Needle holder. A toothed instrument to hold a curved needle for sewing tissue.

Neurons. Nerve cells.

Obligate anaerobic bacteria. Bacteria that grow only in the absence of oxygen. Tetanus and gas gangrene are the most common affecting human beings. A deep puncture wound will seal over and leave tetanus bacteria to grow in the depths away from air.

Osteoblasts. Young connective tissue cells that mature into bony callus.

Outside scrub. Wash-up and shaving of skin around a wound. Done before the wound wash-up.

Palpation. Examination by feeling with the hand.

Parenteral. Other than by mouth.

P.C. After meals.

Penile. Relating to the male penis.

Perineum. Pelvic floor; underneath the crotch.

Phagocytosis. The ingestion of bacteria by white blood cells.

Pneumothorax. Free air in the pleural cavity around the lung. Reduces normal negative pressure and inhibits lung expansion on respiratory (breathing) movements.
External Pneumothorax. Caused by penetrating chest wound.
Internal Pneumothorax. Caused by tear in the lung.

P.R.N. When necessary.

Pylorus. Circular sphincter muscle at the junction of the stomach and duodenum.

Rebound tenderness. Tenderness experienced when firm hand pressure upon abdomen is suddenly released. Indicates peritoneal inflammation.

Serum. Liquid portion of blood exclusive of cells.

Spastic paralysis. Paralysis of a limb but muscles are firmly contracted. Seen later on in head injury or stroke.

Subcutaneous. The region of fatty tissue immediately underneath the skin.

Suppository. Any drug so prepared as to be absorbed after insertion into the rectum.

Sutures. Surgical gobbledygook for stitches or thread.

Systemic. Opposite of "local" with regard to body processes, injury, and disease.

Tenderness. Pain experienced when a part of the body is pressed upon.

Glossary

Therapeutic test. Use of treatment to help make a diagnosis.

Therapy. Treatment.

Thigh. Lower extremity from knee to groin.

T.i.d. Three times daily.

Toothed tissue forceps. Tweezers with teeth for holding tissues.

Urinary tract. Kidneys, ureters (tubes from kidneys to bladder), urinary bladder, urethra (tube from bladder to outside). Male has prostate gland and penis. Female has much shorter urethra.

Vasoconstriction. Narrowing or closing down of blood vessels.

Vasodilation. Dilation of blood vessels.

W.N.L. Within Normal Limits. Abbreviation used in describing results of physical examination.

Wound. Any dissolution or break in integrity of the architecture of a body tissue or tissues.
Avulsed. A wound in which a portion of tissue is torn away or so badly mangled that it is dead (devoid of blood supply) and must be removed by debridement.
Crush. A wound in which the force compresses tissue; it may be strong enough to break open the skin and other structures.
Incised. A clean cut as with a knife or other sharp instrument.

Wound wash-out. Actual scrubbing and rinsing the depths of a wound.

Index

Index

Index

Index